Here is just a glimpse of the fascinating material that is discussed — clearly, authoritatively, in full detail — in this book:

HEART SURGERY

Sewing up a heart...patching a heart...removing the heart's cover...heart valve surgery.

DRUGS AND ANTIBIOTICS

Penicillin, its uses in surgery...new antibiotics...the "-mycins."

SURGERY IN WORLD WAR II

How 96 per cent of wounded men were saved...surgery at the front...what we learned.

PLASTIC SURGERY

New noses from ribs...new jaws from shinbones...removal of scars.

HOW SURGERY CURES CANCER

Treatment by operation and female hormones...benign tumors ...surgery in cancer of the breast, skin, lung.

Plus new operations for diabetes, respiratory ailments; on the liver and gall bladder...surgery to control high blood pressure— and much, much more illuminating and up-to-date information.

This book is a completely rewritten version of The New Science of Surgery, *published originally by Julian Messner, Inc.*

SCIENCE

and

SURGERY

by

DR. FRANK G. SLAUGHTER

PERMABOOKS • MONTREAL, P.Q.

This Permabook edition, completely revised and rewritten, is printed from brand-new plates made from newly set, clear, easy-to-read type.

SCIENCE AND SURGERY

PERMABOOK edition published October, 1956
2nd printing......................August, 1957

This book is a completely rewritten version of *The New Science of Surgery,* published originally by Julian Messner, Inc., in 1946.

PERMABOOK editions are published in the United States by Pocket Books, Inc. and in Canada by Pocket Books of Canada, Ltd.—the world's largest publishers and distributors of low-priced books for the entire family.

CONTENTS

Chapter   *Page*

1. Science and Surgery

The dead live—A patch on the heart—Discoveries in other sciences used in surgery   1

2. The Battle Against Shock

Death from shock, wounds, accidents, burns—The tissue-damage theory—The adrenal glands in shock—Welch bacillus—The blood in shock—Red cells and plasma—Blood proteins—Transfusions of whole blood—Treatment by plasma—Dried plasma   6

3. Injecting Sleep

Earliest anesthetics—Chloroform, ether, nitrous oxide—Ethylene, cyclopropane, di-vinyl ether—Barbiturates—Avertin—Injections directly into the blood stream—Pentothal Sodium, its handling and uses—Spinal anesthesia—Caudal injections in childbirth   20

4. God's Powders

Penicillin—Its discovery by Dr. Fleming—Why it was not developed or used for

*many years—Sulfanilamide—Uses in con-
nection with surgery—Its limitations—
Sulfapyridine—Sulfathiazole—Sulfadiazine
—Penicillin, isolating and producing it
for wide use—What it does—New antibiotics—The "-mycins"*   32

5. Laboratory for War

*Surgery in World War II—96 per cent
of wounded saved—Surgery in previous
wars—Dr. Winnet Orr—Dr. Trueta in the
Spanish Civil War—Gas gangrene—Taking surgery to the front—Welch bacillus
in wounds—Closed plaster treatment—Applications of war to peacetime surgery*   44

6. Peritonitis: The Conquest of a Scourge

*What causes peritonitis—Old treatments
—The Miller-Abbott tube—Blood proteins
in peritonitis—Sulfa drugs and antibiotics
—Other abdominal operations—Need of
plasma*   58

7. Proteins and Prothrombin

*The liver and its functions—The gall blad-
der—Gallstones and surgery—Vitamin K
and clotting of blood—Production of prothrombin—Surgery of the liver and gall
bladder*   69

8. Sweetbreads and Sugar Tolerance

*The pancreas, its double life—The islands
of Langerhans—Diabetes—Insulin—Operating on diabetics—Excess insulin—Tumor*

Chapter *Page*

*of the pancreas—Cancer of the pancreas
meant sure death twenty years ago—The
delicate operation used now—Grafting
pancreatic tissue into diabetics—Transplanting of complete organs* 81

9. **Chest Surgery Comes of Age**

*Surgery and medicine in respiratory infec-
tions—Sucking wounds—Needles and
drains—Anesthesia in modern chest surgery—Intratracheal tubes—Removal of entire lung* 91

10. **Heart Surgery**

*The inside of the heart—Thrombosis and
heparin in heart surgery—Dicoumarin—
Cardiac tamponade—Sewing up a heart
wound—Pericarditis in pneumonia and
rheumatic infection—Removing the heart's
cover—Congenital heart disease in children—Hypothermia—Heart-valve surgery* 103

11. **Saving Limbs with Surgery**

*Vascular surgery, one of the greatest con-
tributions of war to peacetime medicine—
The circulatory system and the autonomic
nervous system—Severance of major blood
vessels no longer means amputation—Vitallium splints for injured blood vessels—
Pulsating hematoma and aneurysm—New,
drastic operations* 116

12. **Life Suspends at Zero**

Crymotherapy, treatment by cold—Refrig-

Chapter   *Page*

> *eration anesthesia—Gangrene in diabetes
> and hardening of the arteries—Experi-
> ments with rats' tails—Effects of cold on
> tissues—Ice saves limbs—Trench foot—
> Other new uses of cold therapy—Can life
> be suspended by cold?*   127

13. Varicose Veins

> *Wide incidence of varicose veins, with
> ulcers, and eczema—How they develop—
> Heredity—Treatment by injections—Dan-
> gers of phlebitis—The operation for vari-
> cose veins*   137

14. Making Operations Safe

> *Safety of surgery today—Remaining dan-
> gers—Pulmonary embolus—Treatment—X-
> rays and venography*   148

15. Wake Up and Walk

> *Brain surgery—Types of skull injuries—
> The spine and the meninges—Operations
> for hemorrhage inside the skull—Blood
> pressure in brain troubles—Spinal punc-
> ture—Treatment by dehydration—Open
> head wounds no longer fatal—Early am-
> bulation in head injuries*   160

16. Psychosurgery

> *Removal of frontal lobe of brain, effects
> on mental illness—Severing of pathways
> from frontal lobe—Moniz' operation—
> American variations—Resulting personali-
> ty changes—Mental illnesses in which sur-*

*gery is not indicated—The future of psy-
chosurgery*   171

17. It May Not Be Sciatica

*Causes of sciatica—The sacroiliac joint—
The spinal column and hernia of the in-
tervertebral disc—Operation to cure it—
Similar ailments, bursitis, neuritis*   180

18. Tantalum: The Living Metal

*Early uses of metal in the body, reac-
tions—Gold, silver, aluminum, magnesium,
vanadium, stainless steel—Vitallium for
bone plates, skull plates, replacement of
bile ducts and arteries—Its limitations—
Tantalum molded into thin plates, thin
foil, fine wires—Use in nerve surgery,
tantalum sutures, foil coverings—Tantalum foil on brain tissues—Replacing defects in bones—Covering hernias with metal plates—Tantalum gauze—Tantalum in
plastic surgery*   188

19. Bundling for Burns

*Effects of burns—Tannic-acid treatment,
now largely abandoned—Shock in severe
burns—Plasma—Infection in burns—Surgery and the wonder drugs—New treatment as surgical operations with vaseline
gauze and compression—Early skin graft-
ing*   196

Chapter *Page*

20. New Faces

*Facial and jaw injuries—New strides in
plastic surgery—Wiring of bone fragments
—New noses from ribs—Use of diced
cartilage—Molds from tantalum—New
jaws from shinbones—New lips from scalp
tissue—Removal of scars—Skin grafting—
Elimination of stitches—Thromboplastics
in affixing new skin—Whole-skin grafts
from leg or abdomen—Replacement of
muscles—New skin over jaws, new gums—
Artificial replacements—Control of fingers
on artificial hands* 208

21. Psychology for Surgeons

*Emotions and their influence on disease—
Autonomic nervous system again—Digestive tract especially susceptible—Ulcers—
Nervous colitis—When psychiatry supplants surgery* 218

22. Surgery Cures Cancer

*Cures by X-ray and radium—Potentialities
of atom-splitting in creating new radioactive substances for cancer treatment—
How cancers develop—Cancer of the
breast—The lymphatic vessels and secondary cancer growths—Cancer of the prostate gland, treatment by operation and
female hormones—Benign tumors—Where
cancers grow—Heredity in cancer—Cancer of the skin, of the stomach, intestines, rectum, uterus, cervix, lung, pancreas—Surgery in these cases* 227

Chapter   *Page*

23. **Why Surgery is Expensive**

   *Good surgery quite costly or entirely
   free—Finances of hospitals—Charity work
   by surgeons—The cost of making a surgeon—Surgeons' incomes—How to locate
   a good surgeon—Clinics—Hospitals*   241

24. **Medicine in the Atomic Age**

   *Almost complete control of medical dis-
   eases—Increase in degenerative diseases—
   A population of older people—New medical specialty, geriatrics—New discoveries
   to be expected—Increasing importance of
   endocrine glands, hormones—The question of socialized medicine—Hospital insurance—Group clinics*   249

25. **A Plan for Medical Care**

   *Group Medicine, with some form of pre-
   payment insurance*   259

SCIENCE
AND
SURGERY

1.

SCIENCE AND SURGERY

The dead live—A patch on the heart—Discoveries in other sciences used in surgery

"Nothing is certain except death and taxes," according to an old proverb. Yet such is the sweeping march of events in the Atomic Age that even those seemingly immutable realities no longer hold true. In Florida, homesteads valued at less than $5,000 are exempt from all property taxes. And in a Philadelphia Hospital only a few months ago, a woman lay for fifty minutes on the operating table with no pulse and no heartbeat—the usual criteria of death—yet lived again. Today surgeons put patches on hearts routinely, in an operation unheard of a decade ago; they open that vital organ under direct vision to slit scarred valves and repair defects. The early treatment of wounded in the Korean conflict, using helicopter transport directly from the battlefield, bettered even the lifesaving record of over 96 per cent established in World War II.

Miracles like these aren't exactly commonplace yet, of course, but they illustrate the vast distances that surgical science has covered in the past decades, with the speeded up pace brought about by war, declared and undeclared, and the chilling realities of the Atomic Age. All these achievements are the offspring of a brilliant marriage, the union of science and surgery.

But what has science to do with surgery? Surgery means trained fingers, shining instruments, an amphitheater tense with the drama of life and death, the hush that falls over the audience as the surgeon's hands—trained hands in smooth

1

white rubber gloves—lift the scalpel, and balancing life and death between skilled fingers, make the quick, ruthless cut that brings away a malignant tumor, then suture up spurting blood vessels.

Yes, surgery is all this. Without the skill of the surgeon's fingers, there would be no surgery, no lives saved. But without science there would be no way for that skill to operate.

Take, for example, the operation of putting a patch on the heart. It began with a coronary attack, the sudden blocking of one of the heart's own blood vessels. Such attacks not infrequently come to those who work under a great deal of stress, people whose coronaries are in a continual state of tension from the barrage of nerve impulses that govern the size of the arteries and veins, which form an intricate network throughout the body that doctors call the vascular bed.

Sometimes there are warning signs—pain in the chest and left arm, discomfort in the upper abdomen (often mistaken for gall-bladder disease). The attack is sudden and sharp, the pain lancinating, the collapse profound and complete, a dramatic and terrifying thing to watch. Often the victim dies on the spot. Old-time doctors used to call it "acute indigestion," and it was common talk that one did not survive a third attack. Modern heart specialists know that in this they were right, if their reasoning was wrong. Few patients *do* survive a third severe coronary attack.

The blocking of the coronary artery by spasm and clot is only the beginning of a series of events that may follow a severe coronary attack. Slowly, over a period of weeks, there develops an area of heart muscle that has been weakened by damage to its blood supply. The muscle fibers may grow thin, fray out; the wall gradually yields to a pressure of blood surging against it at each heartbeat. Looking at such a heart in a fluoroscope, the specialist sees a localized bulging of the heart wall in the injured area, thrusting out with each contraction of the heart. Then one day the wall ruptures and all is over.

For years heart specialists looked at such bulging heart walls, the "aneurysms of the heart" that sometimes occurred after coronary damage. There was nothing to be done, they knew. Surgeons couldn't graft a new heart wall, and nothing short of that would strengthen the weakened area.

Then one day a surgeon watched just such a case under the fluoroscope. The story was the same; a coronary attack, severe, the patient barely pulling through. And then an aneurysm of the heart. But this time there was a difference. The surgeon was a specialist in heart surgery, a man who thought in terms of using the scalpel to help injured and diseased hearts.

To this surgeon the bulging, weakened heart posed a problem—not in how long the patient would live or how best to break the news to the family but in whether it was possible to splint that damaged muscle and protect the weakened spot. He thought something could be done, felt confident enough to attempt the operation, and most important of all, possessed the necessary skill and was backed up by modern scientific knowledge and discovery.

The operation succeeded. A patch of tough fascia was successfully placed over a bulging, paper-thin aneurysm of the heart wall. The patient lived five weeks, then died of a coincident infection, but the heart patch held firmly and did not give way. Dr. Claude Beck, of Cleveland, Ohio, a pioneer in heart surgery, had achieved the distinction of another "first" in surgery, the first operation to place a patch on the heart. A dozen sciences stood back of that operation, however. Take away almost any of them and there would have been failure. Working together with the surgeon's skill they spelled success.

The coronary attack was first evidenced by a rising, then falling blood pressure and a diminution in the strength of the heart sounds. Perhaps this was first heard by that amazing instrument, the phonocardiogram, which seeks out and records the tiniest changes in the heart sounds, changes imperceptible to the ear listening with the old-fashioned stethoscope. Electronics were working for the doctor!

The electrocardiograph is invaluable in diagnosing changes in the heart. A sensitive galvanometer, it picks up currents so faint that they would never register on ordinary instruments, yet records them faithfully on a strip of photographic film. Electricity and photography joining to save lives!

The fluoroscope utilizes physics—the ability of X-rays, generated in a vacuum tube and consisting of a stream of ultrasmall electrons, to activate certain chemicals in a fluoroscopic screen until a glowing picture of the heart and its action appears. Electronics again, but doing the same work!

Before an operation, too, it is necessary to know the exact status of the patient's general condition, best shown by examinations of the blood. The hemoglobin values are measured by the color intensity of iron pigments released from red blood cells, to determine the blood's oxygen-carrying power. The blood-sugar level, nitrogen level, protein determinations, and estimations of the calcium, phosphorus, uric acid, urea—all are determined by chemical reactions, which frequently are finally read by means of the photoelectric colorimeter. An amazing adaptation of the science of optics to chemical observation!

At the operation itself, science stands always at the elbow of the surgeon. Air-conditioned operating rooms prevent undue loss of fluid by evaporation and by direct escape from open body cavities. Ultraviolet lamps suspended from the ceiling fill the air with a faint tinge of ozone and the reddish glow of invisible light, implementing the discovery made years ago that ultraviolet light in very low concentration can effectively kill bacteria in the air, thus preventing infections in operative wounds.

The anesthetist adjusts his machine. Chemistry and physics discovered cyclopropane, the gas that can be given with 80 per cent oxygen, a definite advantage to a patient who must breathe with only one lung during an operation in which the chest may be open for hours. Medicine men in the South American jungles gave us curare, which has been refined by pharmacology, the science of drugs, to a potent anesthetic aid. Physics, too, studied the pressure changes inside the chest and adapted an anesthetic machine to produce the slightly elevated pressure necessary to inflate the lung and prevent dangerous collapse.

Beside the table hangs a flask of blood. Physiological chemists learned long ago that a harmless citrate solution prevents blood from clotting, making transfusion a simple procedure. Now a new drug, heparin, does the same thing.

The shock the blood seeks to prevent depends upon a physicochemical change, a complicated process involving those giant molecules called colloids, their chemistry and their physical characteristics, and the biological phenomena of osmotic pressure and semipermeable membranes, familiar to every college student of biology. And always ready at the surgeon's side when needed are ACTH and cortisone, the powerful new hormones that have revolutionized so many phases of medical science.

Over the surgeon's head is a powerful light that casts no shadow, generates no heat. A system of lenses and mirrors bathes the operating field with a glow of shadowless light.

After the operation is completed, an oxygen tent waits. An electric pump fills the tent and removes the expired air, forcing it through a canister of soda lime, which removes the carbon dioxide by a chemical change and sends pure oxygen back into the tent. Protecting the patient against infection, too, are the sulfa drugs, penicillin, and the newest of all God's Powders, the "-mycin" group.

From this same combination of science and surgery will come the discoveries of the future: the cure of cancer; new techniques in the fight against peritonitis; developments in that newest field, vascular surgery, now on the very threshold of its individual place in science; fuller knowledge of crymotherapy, treatment by cold; and many other innovations not yet envisioned.

Wherever the surgeon performs his miracles with the scalpel, there is Science, always at his elbow, unseen, unheard, but as active an agent in saving lives as the surgeon's own fingers.

This is a small part of the absorbing story of the new science of surgery at the dawning of that magic era, the Atomic Age. The whole story will never be written, for new discoveries make others old before they reach print; but what has been done makes a saga as thrilling as any ever recounted. It begins with the story of three great conquests, without which surgical science would have been powerless to continue its progress—the conquests of shock, of pain, and of infection.

2.

THE BATTLE AGAINST SHOCK

Death from shock, wounds, accidents, burns—
The tissue-damage theory—The adrenal glands
in shock—Welch bacillus—The blood in shock—
Red cells and plasma—Blood proteins—Trans-
fusions of whole blood—Treatment by plasma—
Dried plasma

In World War I thousands of wounded soldiers died, but not from wounds themselves. They died from a strange, then only half-understood by-product of the wound that, for lack of a better term, we call "shock." Brought down on the battlefield, they lay sometimes for hours on the cold ground, in the damp, frosty air of France, often in a cold drizzle. Generally, if they were alive on arrival at the first temporary hospital, the picture was much the same, no matter what the wound.

These casualties were pale, often actually blue, from oxygen-lack—the determining factor in prognosis in such cases. Their pulses were racing to keep up a rapidly failing circulation. Their blood pressure was very low, and the tips of their fingers and toes, if not already blue from oxygen-lack and cold, appeared entirely devoid of blood. They weren't unconscious, as a rule—not until just before the end, sometimes not until the very end itself. And those were deaths that seared the nerves of doctors, because they were completely impotent to help; they knew nothing really about this lethal process that sapped away lives they could easily have saved had it been only the wounds that needed treatment.

What little those front-line doctors could do they did,

working in dugouts or old, abandoned buildings. The patients were cold; they gave them warmth. They piled on blankets to conserve body heat, and they added internal warmth in the form of hot drinks to those who could take them. They rigged up lamps and other ingenious devices to apply external heat. Sometimes they saw almost miraculous things occur with heat alone, but often there was little if any effect. All recognized that they were dealing with a change that at some point became irreversible. After that, nothing did any good.

They weren't entirely unaccustomed to this picture, those civilian surgeons turned medical soldiers for the duration. They had seen it before in accident cases and in surgical operations that were difficult and long drawn out. They'd seen it particularly in hemorrhage cases and in severe burns, but they recognized that shock was not the result of mere loss of blood. Sometimes the blood loss was negligible but the shock was severe, even fatal.

And so when the first great conflict ended, these medical-school professors turned military doctors went back to their practices, their laboratories, their classrooms. Some things they had noted, as trained observers should, on the battlefield. One of these—perhaps the most important, for in it lay the clue to solving the whole problem—was simple. In those bad shock cases, especially toward the end, a strange thing happened to the blood. Somehow it became thick; it no longer flowed freely from cut blood vessels but was actually thick, almost too viscid to flow through the blood vessels themselves.

With the thickness came another change, equally obvious: the blood was dark, almost black. The thickness they couldn't understand, for in many cases there had been no actual loss of blood from the circulation, no hemorrhage. They could name it—they called it hemoconcentration—but they couldn't entirely understand it.

Explaining the darkness was simple. Fresh blood, leaving the lungs with plenty of vital oxygen in it, is bright red. As it loses oxygen to tissue cells in an incredibly rapid chemical change, whereby "oxyhemoglobin," the red coloring matter of the red blood cells, becomes "reduced hemoglobin," it changes in color, becomes darker, less red. Obviously this thick blood in shock cases was oxygen-poor blood. The corollary to this observation was that death in shock cases came from oxygen-lack to the hair-trigger-sensitive cells of the vital centers of the brain. But it was many years before this conclusion could be reached.

Shock demanded much of the attention of medical-research scientists after World War I, for shock was universal in severe accidents, whether military or civilian. And with the growing use of mechanical appliances like the automobile, more civilized methods of killing themselves, or at least maiming their bodies, were being put into the hands of people every day. Being scientists as well as doctors, they approached this problem in a scientific manner, by searching for the cause.

And right there they ran into a snag, for even now, with all we know about shock and with everything we have developed to treat it once it occurs, we don't really understand what causes it. We know the kind of case in which it will occur, and we can institute treatment that often prevents it from actually developing. Certainly we can keep it from getting ahead of us except in a small percentage of cases in which nothing seems to have any effect. But what the actual mechanism is that produces shock—that, with all our scientists, our marvelously intricate scientific instruments, our thousands of investigators working in laboratories, we still haven't discovered.

Military and civilian surgeons had noticed a few other things, too, in addition to the oxygen-lack and increased viscidity of the blood. One was that shock tended to develop in crushing types of injuries, those in which the essential feature seemed to be injury to muscle tissue. Reasoning logically, they postulated a substance derived from injured muscles that, absorbed into the body, caused the startling changes in circulation that gave the shock picture.

For a while this tissue-damage theory held sway, and in a way it was a good thing. For, if incorrect—as it most probably is—it did engender in surgeons' minds a healthy respect for muscle-tissue damage, and it made them "no-further-injury" conscious. They set about teaching people to let broken bones lie until someone with a splint or stretcher could reach the scene, instead of picking up a broken leg and moving it around, jamming broken bone ends into the flesh and increasing the damage already present. Emphasis was placed on splinting fractures early, and the American College of Surgeons put out a simple little manual called a *Primer on Fractures* so the average doctor didn't need to be a bone specialist to know how to handle a broken bone properly. And they began to try to standardize treatment of many traumatic injuries (that's a long word meaning injuries from external causes, or simply, accidents, ranging from sunburn to torn limbs).

Doctors hadn't learned the cause of shock yet, but they were a long way toward keeping it from being aggravated once the injured person was reached by someone trained enough in first aid to start the correct treatment.

The muscle-crush theory didn't explain shock, although some investigators still think it may play a part, so these scientists went on to other theories. They even searched for the cause in the ubiquitous little glands located right above the kidneys, called the adrenals. Already they knew that a powerful substance was produced by the central portion of those glands, a substance called adrenalin, which exerted a marvelously stimulating effect on the heart and often brought quick relief to asthma sufferers. There was an outer layer to this gland, too, and here they searched for something that might explain shock.

It wasn't just hit-or-miss experimentation, either. One disease, we know, is due to a deficiency of that cortex, a slowly fatal illness called Addison's disease. Characterizing it, among other things, is a remarkable weakness and a lowering of the blood pressure. Shock lowered blood pressure, *ergo*, they might be related. And strangely enough it really looked as if they might, for the potent extract of the adrenal cortex did exert a stimulating effect on shock patients. Series of cases were injected with this cortical extract or hormone, and often the results were gratifying.

Now, with the Atomic Age miracles of ACTH and cortisone, we know that the hormones of the adrenal cortex are powerful aids in treating early shock, sometimes lifesaving, in fact. But disturbances of these are not the cause, that's certain.

This wasn't the whole story, though, for in intestinal obstruction, when the bowel becomes distended with gas and fluid and the patient rapidly becomes toxic, a picture closely resembling true shock often occurs. This didn't at all fit the conception that shock was of traumatic origin, and so the researchers went back to work. They studied the contents of these distended intestines and found them teeming with malignant germs, particularly the Welch bacillus of gas gangrene. The toxic poison of the Welch bacillus was isolated, and for a while it was believed to be the cause of shock in those obstruction cases. That theory, too, had its period of favor only to be discarded.

While they were investigating the cause, making false starts but always learning something from every new tack, scientists were also investigating the treatment of shock. And here they made rapid strides. The World War I observation of thick blood was studied thoroughly, using new instruments, chemical analysis of the blood to determine which of its constituents actually was lost, and replacement therapy to try to bring shocked blood back to its normal concentration.

In the laboratory one thing became obvious. What seemed to be thick blood was really thick blood—thick because the red cells, comprising about half its volume, stayed in the circulation while the fluid portion of the blood, in which the cells floated, diminished. The difficult thing was to determine where the fluid went when it left the blood stream. That required further investigation and a thorough study of the constitution of the blood. The results were definite and important; they are the basis for our modern treatment of shock, which is saving such a high percentage of wounded in war and in civilian trauma.

Blood is really two things. First, there are cells, living cells. The red ones carry hemoglobin and, therefore, oxygen. The white ones, the policemen of the body, attack infection and multiply in the presence of inflammation, giving the high blood counts the surgeon uses in diagnosing appendicitis. Taken together, these cells make up about half the blood volume.

Now, take a sample of blood and mix it with some sodium citrate to keep it from clotting (much as is done now in the process of indirect transfusion, which has changed the transferring of blood from one person to another from a major operation to a simple procedure). Let this mixture settle for a while—or put it in the centrifuge and whirl it at high speed, taking advantage of the fact that the solid, heavier cells will fly outward because of centrifugal force and pack themselves in the bottom of the flask—and the cells can thus be separated from the brownish fluid above them. This fluid is the other constituent of blood, plasma, the more important half as far as shock is concerned.

The scientists didn't stop there in the search for the truths about blood, however. They investigated the construction of this liquid fragment and found that it, too, could be divided into portions. One is entirely fluid, purely chemical—a solution of sodium chloride (ordinary salt) along with some other minerals, such as calcium, which is necessary for the proper clotting of the blood; potassium, which affects the heart muscle so remarkably; and a few other less important elements. These are chemicals, they obey the ordinary chemical laws, and the effect of changes in their concentration can be calculated in advance by any chemist with a slide rule or a logarithm table.

Dissolved in plasma are some other substances, though, less easy to understand. These are proteins, largely belonging to two great groups, the albumens and the globulins. Their complex molecules give blood its sticky characteristic, its viscosity. They aren't simple chemical compounds, these proteins, and their effects can't always be prophesied.

Scientists learned a lot more about these large molecules, called colloids. For one thing, they are ordinarily too large to pass through the walls of the blood vessels. Tending to remain inside the circulation, they exert a peculiar effect called osmotic pressure; that is, when they get too numerous they tend to draw water through the blood-vessel walls and into the circulation. Conversely, when the protein-colloid concentration is too low to maintain the normal amount of water in the circulation, the blood becomes less watery.

But less water means less plasma, and less plasma means an automatic increase in the number of red and white cells per volume unit of blood, for the number of cells do not change. It also means a decrease in the total volume of blood. All that is simple arithmetic, calculable in the laboratory.

What happened to the blood then? This was the question that set researchers talking, hoping that finally they had found the secret of shock. For this less-watery blood was thick and viscid; in short, it was the blood of shock except that there was no change in the oxygen content.

The theory that shock might be tied up with low blood proteins was an interesting one. Best of all it was a theory that proved to be actual fact, an interesting hypothesis that can be simply explained.

This hypothesis said that control of the volume of the circulating blood lay in those protein molecules, called colloids. Given a normal concentration of blood proteins, other things being normal, like the salt content and the waste products being carried to the kidneys, there would be a normal amount of water dissolving that protein—*ergo*, a normal blood volume. But lower the protein in the blood and the water-pulling power—scientifically described by the term "colloid osmotic pressure"—diminished. Water couldn't be held in the circulation; it escaped into the tissues, and if the blood proteins got too low, swelling developed in the ankles, about the eyes, perhaps all over the body. The water balance was simply out of kilter, and nothing could adjust it except replacing those lowered blood proteins.

That's why surgeons, pumping salt solution into postoperative patients because they couldn't take fluids by mouth, found the salt escaping into the tissues, causing swelling and preventing the proper healing of wounds. That's why medical men found that cases of malnutrition, such as children who did not get the proper amount of protein food and adults who suffered from long and debilitating illnesses, often got swollen feet and ankles.

Most important of all was the likelihood that here was the explanation of shock. It required only a simple corollary to prove to the satisfaction of many doctors that it really happened this way. That corollary was the idea of "increased capillary permeability." What did that mean? Simply that under certain conditions, notably from crushing wounds, from exposure, or from a distended bowel with intestinal obstruction, the walls of the capillaries, the blood vessels that surround every cell in the body, changed somehow. Now instead of keeping the huge protein molecules inside the blood vessels, maintaining the normal colloid osmotic pressure and keeping the normal amount of water in the volume of the circulating blood, the damaged capillary walls allowed them to escape into the areas around the cells, the tissue spaces. So the protein content was lowered and the blood became thicker.

From there on it was easy to figure what was happening. Thick blood being harder to pump, the heart worked faster to get it around the circulation. Result, a rapid pulse. The volume of blood was sharply cut by this loss through the capillary walls; therefore, the pressure in the entire pumping system fell. Result, a lowered blood pressure. But this the body wouldn't take without a fight, for falling blood pressure means a failing circulation to the brain.

The brain looks after itself, for it knows that it cannot long stand a failing circulation with a lowering of the amount of oxygen brought to it from the lungs. The great automatic nervous system of the body—the system that controls vital functions like respiration, digestion, and circulation without our ever becoming conscious that they are functioning until they get out of rhythm—sets to work. It can't increase the blood volume; therefore, it decreases the length and size of the pipeline. All over the body, tiny nerves running along the blood vessels go into action, shrinking the vessels, shutting some of them off altogether, carrying out a marvelously complicated operation we summarize with two words, *peripheral vasoconstriction*.

That's why the shocked patient's hands and feet are pale: blood has been shunted from them to the central circulation of the body, preserving to the very last the integrity of the blood supply to the brain. Temporarily, under this influence, the blood pressure is boosted in an attempt to maintain normal circulation. The pulse is rising, but the blood pressure rises a little, too. An untrained observer might be fooled, might not realize the significance of those pale, cyanotic hands and feet, the rapid pulse, the hurried breathing to provide a maximum supply of blood through the lungs.

Doctors recognized that this was the time to carry out treatment to prevent this process from going any further, so it was vital for this period to be recognized before disaster took place.

Draw a chart of the pulse and the blood pressure in a severely injured patient, check them every few minutes, and plot the lines. They go up together—to a point. There the increased pulse rate and the decrease in the size of the circulation trying to accommodate itself to the diminished blood volume get out of balance. Some observers call this the "critical point."

What happens after this? If proper treatment is not carried out rapidly—and sometimes in spite of any treatment—the pressure starts falling, the blood fails to get its proper supply of oxygen, the nervous system begins to be affected (for nerve cells are extremely sensitive to changes in their oxygen supply), and serious oxygen-lack begins to make itself evident by the dark color of the blood. Then comes a release of the protecting tension of the tiny blood vessels, the entire circulation fails—and death.

How to discover this process early enough to reverse it? That was the problem medical scientists labored over. Knowing its presence, they could do much to combat it. Injecting fluids into the circulation helped temporarily, not always permanently, for without enough protein in the blood to hold the fluid, it soon escaped from the circulation. Injecting a colloid-resembling compound called acacia was sometimes of lifesaving value. It stayed in the circulation and held water, to a certain extent, but later it appeared in the liver and no one could be quite certain that it would not injure that delicate organ. Another substance called pectin seemed to have much the same properties. A hundred or more substances were suggested, even tried. Along with these the powerful extract of the adrenal cortex was shot into the veins. Blood pressures usually rose, at least temporarily, and the patients improved. Who could say exactly what did it?

The temporary respite afforded by such stopgap measures gave time in which to match the injured person for a transfusion and shoot into his veins the one thing that could be counted on to stay there, blood. Frequent blood transfusion was the best thing to bulwark circulations failing from shock, and to replace blood lost from hemorrhage. That much had been learned in the battle against shock.

First, however, doctors had to discover the shock early enough to treat it. There they showed their ingenuity, those scientists studying shock, by measuring the blood proteins to determine exactly whether they were normal, low, or high.

A method of doing it was known, a long, involved, time-consuming process of treating the blood with various chemicals, firing it in a long-necked Kjeldahl flask, and finally reading the figures off on a colorimeter. It took a well-equipped laboratory and one that did these examinations frequently, to get dependable results. Meanwhile, the patient might be progressing into deeper stages of shock, from protein-lack. So another group used the idea of measuring the percentage of cells by whirling the blood in a hematocrit tube in a centrifuge until the cells settled down to the bottom. It was an improvement and it didn't take too long, but the results weren't entirely satisfactory. Something better was needed.

Then came along an ingenious little device called a "falling-drop apparatus." The principle is simple. Drop a lead shot and a nut of the same size in a glass of water. The shot plummets to the bottom because it is heavy; the nut descends slowly, if at all, because it is very much lighter. Change the water to oil or any more viscid liquid and the shot drops more slowly because of the resistance, as does the nut. Now drop another pair of objects, but this time exactly equal droplets of a heavy liquid and a light one. Watch them descend, time them for an equal distance, and if you know the weight, the specific gravity, of one of them, you can calculate that of the other.

The falling-drop apparatus is as simple as that. A drop of blood descends through a column of resistant liquid. The time of its fall is recorded and the specific gravity calculated by means of tables.

It's so simple that in many hospitals the apparatus rides around the ward on a cart called the "shock cart." Blood-protein concentrations are calculated right at the bedside. No time is lost by long chemical processes, not even spinning in a centrifuge. In a few moments the surgeon knows whether this patient is developing dangerous protein-lack from loss of plasma through his capillaries or from wounded or burned tissues. A few minutes more and he is taking the logical steps to correct this lack.

And there's the story of shock. Find it early, and treat it adequately. It sounds simple and it is, in principle, but a lot had to be done yet. How best to replace this protein loss? Blood did it, surgeons knew, but in some cases, notably severe burns, there was a marked protein loss, and every time lost plasma was added with blood, more red blood cells were also added. They weren't needed at all; they only served to thicken the already too thick blood. A few transfusions were fine, but if this plasma-replacement treatment was to be kept up, some way had to be found to get rid of those red cells.

The answer was simple: once the lost blood was replaced by transfusion, give only the plasma, leaving the cells behind. The two could be separated in the laboratory to obtain specimens of plasma; it remained only to do so on a large scale, a trifling problem for scientific ingenuity that could dream up an intricate little piece of apparatus like the falling-drop machine.

It worked out like this. Take the blood, mix it with citrate, let the cells settle out—or better still, whirl it in a centrifuge— until they are packed at the bottom of the bottle. Then siphon off the clear, brownish plasma, add a little antiseptic to preserve it, stopper it tightly, and there is a bottle of plasma ready to be taken wherever it is needed. With a lot of donors, the plasma from all of them is mixed together so as to dilute any tendency one man's blood might have to cause reactions. Fortunately, plasma can be given without having to be matched, for most of the difficulty in matching blood for transfusions is in getting the red cells of the two people to agree.

That, of course, was a long step, the greatest step yet taken in the treatment of shock. Doctors still weren't sure exactly what went on to cause the protein loss, but they knew how to recognize it. And they knew how to treat it, by replacing lost protein with liquid plasma. But there were a few things yet to trouble medical investigators. Liquid plasma couldn't be stored too long, a couple of years at most. And it couldn't be used in extreme heat or cold. Too much heat and it went bad, too much cold and it froze and was no good. The perfect replacement fluid needed to be capable of use anywhere.

The serum manufacturers had the answer to that. Years before, they had perfected a method of making serums for pneumonia, scarlet fever, and tetanus, all the hundreds of protective agents they manufactured, in a new form, as solids. They did this by evaporating the water out of the serum, leaving behind the proteins, which are the active agents. Serums lasted longer this way, they found, and were easier to handle. It was only necessary to inject a little water back into the ampule containing the brownish-white powder and instantly the serum was ready for injection.

Handling blood plasma that way was good business for the manufacturers. Many people would rather pay for the commercial plasma than go through the process of getting donors in, taking the blood, separating the plasma, and making it ready for injection. And besides, not many hospitals could afford the apparatus necessary for a plasma bank. So manufacturers worked out a simple method of plasma concentration, first by freezing, then quickly evaporating in a vacuum. Soon ampules of dried blood plasma began to appear on the market, selling for about the amount ordinarily paid a professional blood donor for a transfusion.

They saved thousands of lives, those ampules of dried blood plasma. They were used everywhere during World War II. Into the very foxholes they went, bringing protection from shock to every wounded man who needed it. Unfortunately, with mass production from millions of donors, some unwelcome visitors managed to creep in. Most dangerous of these was the virus of hepatitis, commonly called jaundice, a pretty bad actor in some cases. Many people carry this virus around in their blood for years without knowing they have it. But injected into someone else, it can cause serious effects; in fact, hepatitis was one of the big headaches of World War II.

Now ways have been discovered to exterminate the persistent hepatitis virus. It's done most effectively in one of two ways. One way is to irradiate all plasma with ultraviolet light, which seems to take care of the virus. The other is to keep the plasma pools in small amounts, say eight to ten donor-batches, at room temperature for six months. After that, the hepatitis bugs seem to give up the ghost.

A lot of trouble? Not at all. Nothing is too much trouble when a human life is at stake. Remember that the next time you have a chance to give blood at your local blood bank.

Science had discovered a way to identify shock, and a way to treat it that seemed foolproof, but it didn't stop there. Two types of proteins occur in blood plasma, albumen and globulin. Globulin isn't very important in shock, although it is apparently the medium in which lies the protection of the antibodies we develop when we're vaccinated against smallpox, diphtheria, typhoid, and similar diseases. Until the development of the Salk vaccine, immune globulin taken from people who had developed a certain amount of resistance to poliomyelitis, seemed to be the only form of protection we had against that scourge. Now, fortunately, the vaccine seems to hold out promise of exterminating this disease.

It is the serum albumen that is really important as a water-holding protein in the blood. Now it has been separated from the globulin so that the protein from an ordinary transfusion can be injected from an ampule the doctor can hold in the palm of his hand. An injection can be given practically anywhere in this way, and the albumen has proved tremendously valuable in controlling the dangerous head pressure that develops after brain operations or injuries on some occasions.

War injuries proved something surgeons knew already, that any severely injured person is best treated with real blood. Plasma serves well as a stopgap, even in cases of hemorrhage, but if important surgery is to be performed, the patient needs whole blood, the best stimulant yet found. Front-line hospital workers gave blood generously in the early stages of World War II, but that was not sufficient. If too much was taken from these eager donors, their efficiency was impaired, and this only hindered their work. A method of getting large quantities of blood into the front areas had to be devised.

Here, too, scientists were working in the Army Medical Center, in the Navy Medical Center, and in medical schools all over the world. One thing they knew: generally it is safe to give blood belonging to Type O, the Universal Donor, to anyone without matching. And something like a third of the people were this type. Also, they knew that blood placed at low temperatures could be kept for many days. With these facts in hand, it didn't take long to work out a feasible procedure.

The blood of some Type O donors, instead of being used to make plasma, was placed in a special container, tested, chilled, and flown overseas. Still in its original bottle, it was rushed up front and injected into the veins of a wounded man, building up his strength for a necessary operation. Sixteen thousand such pint bottles of blood were used on Iwo Jima alone.

The story of blood and blood substitutes in shock is far from finished. Every month new progress is reported in the medical journals. Shock isn't licked yet, but we're in the last rounds of the battle—and we're winning. Meanwhile, there are other fields in which this story of progress through science needs to be told. One of the foremost of these is in anesthesia.

3.

INJECTING SLEEP

Earliest anesthetics—Chloroform, ether, nitrous oxide—Ethylene, cyclopropane, di-vinyl ether—Barbiturates—Avertin—Injections directly into the blood stream—Pentothal Sodium, its handling and uses—Spinal anesthesia—Caudal injections in childbirth

Since ancient times man has sought for the perfect anesthetic agent. The requirements of this ideal substance were simple. It must be safe, pleasant to use, and effective, bringing the unconsciousness so necessary for the surgeon to perform his miracles of the scalpel, yet causing no ill effects to the patient and minimum unpleasantness in both entering and leaving the unconscious state. Ancient physicians had no anesthesia, save the pain-soothing effects of opium and alcohol, neither effective enough to permit painless surgery and both dangerous if used to the point of deep unconsciousness. They may have been conscious of the anesthetic effect of cold, but no definite records of its use are available. Some pinned their faith on sleep-producing draughts of herbal extracts; some merely shut their ears to the screams of their patient and operated without anesthesia until unconsciousness brought him surcease from pain.

In the early portions of the last century a few courageous doctors began to use a new and pungent chemical compound that seemed for a while to be the answer to the problem. Certainly in chloroform they had the nearest to a perfect anesthetic that had ever been used. It was not too unpleasant, although its pungent odor could not be termed attractive. It was rapid in its action—too rapid sometimes, for the patient might drop into the critical deeper stages of anesthesia before the person administering the vapor recognized the danger.

But there were also dangerous side effects of chloroform, not known then but definitely proved now. Most important was its effect on the liver. Case after case crossed autopsy tables with livers shrunken and pale, the deep brown of bile pigment changed to the light color of liver damage, designated by the pathologists as "yellow atrophy."

At first the doctors couldn't understand this change, could not pin down the culprit as the pain-destroying chloroform, although some suspected it. Many people took chloroform without suffering liver damage, and even now we cannot tell who will be hurt by it. But the possibility of such a life-endangering change in the vital functions of the liver made widespread use of chloroform too dangerous. It enjoyed an era of popularity, in which it even achieved the royal distinction of being designated "anaesthesia à la reine" because it was reputed to have been used during the *accouchement* of an English queen.

Even this era was not without its moments of turbulence, however, for the pain-relieving properties of chloroform in its then favorite use, to allay the agonies of childbirth, were attacked by the clerics as immoral and against the teachings of the Scriptures. This period of intolerance when the baby science of anesthesia fought to achieve its rightful place as a branch of the healing art, is just another example of the way in which small reactionary minorities have always sought to delay the progress of that which is new and untried in science, whether astronomy or zoology.

Consider Galileo and his quarrels with the theories of long-dead Aristotle. Read the storm of abuse and recrimination heaped upon the head of luckless Darwin because he was first to read in the world about us irrefutable signs of the progress that has brought the human race to the present level of development. Then search out the record of the stormy times when Simpson, Semmelweis, and Holmes fought for their theories which were to save thousands of mothers from death in childbirth. All succeeded, but only in spite of relentless opposition.

Opposition can never completely shut away the searching ray of science in quest of knowledge, however, it usually only sharpens the beam and gives it more ultimate penetration. Thus it was inevitable that other substances would be discovered, less dangerous than chloroform yet possessing its undenied anesthetic properties. Two tireless researchers made, almost simultaneously, the same discovery—the fight still goes on to determine which was first—and demonstrated the anesthetic properties of ether to a scoffing and unbelieving medical profession. What does it matter, then, if Crawford Long or Thomas G. Morton was first? The importance of what they did completely transcends any question of personal credit.

Three hundred years after ether was first prepared by Valerius Cordus, the purpose for which it had really been created was demonstrated for the first time. In the hundred years that have followed its discovery, no other anesthetic agent has quite supplanted ether. Even now there are probably more anesthesias carried out with it than with all the other anesthetic agents together. In advanced hospitals of World War I, the old-fashioned ACE mixture, containing chloroform as well as alcohol, was the standard pain-relieving agent while wounds were treated and broken bones strengthened and held in place. Through the years since the war, ether has proved to be the safest anesthetic in the relatively unskilled hands of nurses and student anesthetists.

But ether has its drawbacks, so the search for the perfect anesthetic went on in the laboratories and in the operating rooms throughout the world. Ether, like most volatile agents, causes lung irritation with the production of mucus. It also causes nausea and retching, so patients came to dread the horror of inhaling its pungent fumes. And dreading it, they reacted more violently to it. The reaction was largely one of dread; that was easily proved, for children, who knew nothing of its effects, suffered but little from it. Still there were instances, notably cases involving lung diseases, such as tuberculosis, in which other agents were needed. To cover these drawbacks, many gases were used.

Nitrous oxide, the laughing gas of dentists, is a fine anesthetic agent but the oxygen intake has to be cut down considerably to achieve deep anesthesia with it. Ethylene is more rapid, more pleasant in its action, but possesses fairly high explosiveness. Cyclopropane, a tricky gas requiring the constant attention of a specially trained anesthetist, is probably the nearest to a perfect gas for anesthesia, since it permits the use of exceedingly high percentages of vital oxygen. Unfortunately, cyclopropane is rather highly explosive and so is not so widely used as it would otherwise be. A new derivative of ether called di-vinyl ether, so rapid-acting that a couple of breaths send the patient into dreamland, is widely used as a preliminary agent to remove the choking, struggling period of ether, particularly in tonsil operations and the like.

None of these quite fulfills the requirements of a perfect anesthetic agent, however. Perhaps nothing ever will, for to produce unconsciousness, brain cells must be insulted, and brain cells are very reactive to insult, particularly those of the vital centers controlling the gastrointestinal tract and the vomiting reflex.

Researchers turned to another field, and a new group of drugs came to the fore in the twenties. They were derivatives of a mother compound called barbituric acid, which in turn was one of the multiple offspring of the uninspiring ancestor of so many important medical chemicals—coal tar. They had some desirable properties, those chemicals with complicated formulas. The main one was that they produced sleep, sleep from which the patient would awaken with few if any of the noxious effects of the unconsciousness obtained by older drugs. Also, they were completely destroyed in the body and excreted, instead of remaining for a long time stored in the tissues to exert those unpleasant after-symptoms of headache, nausea, dizziness, and the general effects of a good hangover.

At first the barbiturates weren't entirely innocuous, but chemists were performing daily miracles of synthesis and new compounds were born from coal tar with incredible rapidity. Gradually the new drugs became more rapid in their action and less prolonged in their effects and aftereffects. Preparations were developed that could be injected hypodermically in patients unable to take them by mouth. Medicine's drug-science of pharmacology was making great strides toward the ideal anesthetic agent.

Meanwhile there was a flurry of enthusiasm for a new compound that promised to remove from most volatile anesthetic agents the unpleasant period of induction, when the pungent vapor first strikes the sensitive lining of the respiratory tract. This time it was a derivative of lowly and much maligned alcohol called tribromoethanol, or by the simpler name avertin. Injected in watery solution into the lower bowel as an enema, this drug was absorbed fairly rapidly at first, then more slowly, its effect disappearing after about two and a half hours. Patients liked it, for they went to sleep in their beds, knew nothing of the psychological shock of the trip to the operating room and the anesthetic, and awoke in their own beds once more when the operation was over.

It was nearly a perfect combination—achieving a mild degree of anesthesia in the sickroom and modifying it later, as deeper unconsciousness was necessary, with any one of the gaseous anesthetic agents or with ether. But it had a few drawbacks. One was that the depth of anesthesia couldn't always be controlled; the anesthetist couldn't always predict just how a given case would react. And once injected, the agent was out of control, always a disquieting thought to surgeon and anesthetist alike. Even so, avertin was so much better for its particular uses than anything previously developed that it was widely employed, and still is, as a basal anesthetic.

About this time, near the beginning of the nineteen thirties, a few hardy pioneers began injecting some of the barbiturate compounds directly into the blood stream, putting the anesthetic agent right where it would go to work most effectively. Doctors knew that morphine injected into the blood stream acts immediately, even before the needle can be removed. Sometimes it had to be used this way in an emergency to control the unbearable lancinating pain of kidney colic. It wasn't entirely new, this idea of injecting sleep, but it was just beginning to be recognized as the valuable adjunct to medical practice it is, for the more exacting requirements of the surgeon. Doctors in mental hospitals had long used in emergencies a shot of pungent paraldehyde injected directly into a vein and knew its power to turn a maniacal patient, bent on destroying himself and those about him, into a sleeping babe in a matter of seconds.

Pharmacologists began to try out these barbituric-acid derivatives, drugs that went under chemical names such as phenobarbital and pentobarbital, with formulas that chased each other around rings until an ordinary person got dizzy trying to follow them. The first they tried were too long-acting, their effects too difficult to control, but they went on to use other compounds, each shorter-acting and more easily excreted by the body, either by destruction to less complex substances in the liver or by direct loss through the kidneys.

The first really effective drug for anesthesia by way of the veins was a fine white powder that produced unconsciousness before the anesthetist could remove his needle from the vein. It looked like the perfect agent, and very nearly approached that. But its action was not quite controllable enough to suit conservative anesthetists; they wanted something they could depend on a little better, that they could inject a little more slowly, controlling the level of anesthesia as they went, keeping the patient always just deep enough for the operation but not so deep that he could not be brought out rapidly by ceasing the injection or by using one of the powerful stimulants such as Metrazol, a drug that can snap a patient from unconscious to wide awake in seconds.

And then, working at the Mayo Clinic, pioneer anesthetist Dr. John S. Lundy found the right substance. It didn't look so different from the others. They were white powders, this was yellow, showing that it contained sulfur, which was indicated in its name, thiopentobarbital, shortened soon to pentothal. But it was different. It acted more rapidly, and what was more important, the body got rid of it in a matter of minutes.

Pentothal had to be kept flowing into the circulation at a steady rate to maintain unconsciousness, but this was exactly what the anesthetists wanted. They wanted the patient to go under fast, so fast he didn't have time to worry about what was happening to him. And they wanted him ready to come out again just about as quickly. Pentothal, or rather the sodium salt of the drug, accomplished just those things. After Dr. Lundy had demonstrated in thousands of cases that it was a safe anesthetic agent for many operations that weren't too long and didn't require too deep a sleep, surgeons all over the country began to use it.

Pentothal Sodium is ideal for a lot of things, from opening a boil to setting a broken arm. Some anesthetists use it for serious operations, even abdominal work, especially in conjunction with the more recently perfected agents, such as curare. Like all anesthetic drugs, it exerts a depressive effect on the respiration, and if too much is injected breathing stops. Fortunately, the difference between the point at which respiration ceases and that at which the heartbeat is also stopped, is the mark of a safe anesthetic.

Pentothal belongs to the safe group. One thing the anesthetist can bet on, and it's a comforting thing to know, is that the heart of the patient who gets an overdose will always still be beating if breathing does stop. This means there is ample time to institute artificial respiration and keep things going until the drug can be removed by the liver and the depth of anesthesia lightened. Cessation of breathing is not a particularly comforting thing to have happen; fortunately it's an easy one to control.

Anesthetists in military hospitals estimated that about 80-odd per cent of the operations on wounded men did not require deep surgical anesthesia. What was needed was a rapid-acting anesthetic, one that could be administered in a foxhole if necessary yet from which the patient recovered rapidly with little side effect. Pentothal Sodium filled that bill so completely that in many front-line hospitals very little else was used. It is easy to carry, requiring only one ampule for the powder and another for the water to dissolve it, plus a syringe with which to inject it. It's pleasant for the wounded soldier. He feels the prick of a needle and starts counting aloud. At about the count of twelve he starts to yawn, usually grins, and then snores. Fifteen to thirty seconds from the needle prick he is usually unconscious. A few minutes and he is ready for operation on a compound fracture or a deep flesh wound.

Best of all, the anesthetic injection doesn't interfere with the all-important injection of plasma to control shock. It doesn't even necessitate two needle pricks. If the plasma is already flowing into the veins, the needle of the anesthetic syringe is merely thrust through the rubber tubing of the plasma set and the Pentothal injected directly into the stream of plasma running into the blood current. Under battle conditions, a trained anesthetist can watch enlisted technicians at several operating tables at once, going from one to the other, supervising the injection, and saving manpower at a time when manpower saved means lives saved, too.

But war surgery isn't the only field where Pentothal finds use. In fact, in whatever new place it is used, a new function is usually discovered. Painful dressings, for years the curse of the patient ill for a long time with burns or other wounds, are no more. A few drops of Pentothal put the patient into a state of analgesia or partial sleep, from which he recovers quickly, with the painful period safely behind him.

Even in head wounds, Pentothal, first thought to be contra-indicated, has shown itself a most valuable agent. Increased intracranial pressure, or swelling of the brain, long the anesthesia bugaboo of surgeons treating injured brains, is reduced by Pentothal Sodium. Long series of cases have been reported—including difficult brain operations lasting several hours, the acid test of any anesthetic—and the new injected sleep has come through with colors flying. Deep in the jungle, where tropical heat makes it impossible to use highly volatile ether; in Arctic regions where the frozen water in the ampules has to be melted before the solution can be prepared for injection—in either place it works equally well.

But that doesn't mean that anyone can use Pentothal Sodium; like any anesthetic, it is risky. Inject too fast and the concentration of the drug gets ahead of the effect, causing it to pile up and rapidly increasing the danger of overdosage. Inject without the proper preparation of a hypodermic of morphine and atrophine to control the initial period of throat spasm that sometimes occurs and there's likely to be serious trouble from the start. That's why trained anesthetists went to the front-line hospitals, into the emergency foxhole operating rooms on Pacific beaches, with landing troops in amphibious assault. For wherever surgery is brought to the wounded man, anesthesia must be brought also. Needless pain causes needless increase in shock. Why cause needless pain when it can be prevented in five minutes with an ampule of Pentothal and a syringe?

These are not the only ways of preventing pain at operation. Often it is unnecessary, even inadvisable, to have the patient asleep.

In surgery on patients properly prepared—the kind of surgery done in civilian operating rooms over the country—there is little danger of lowered blood pressure from shock, such as often prevents the use of the nearly perfect spinal anesthesia in abdominal wounds at the front.

Surgeons like spinal anesthesia because it gives perfect relaxation, no worry about danger to the patient's lungs, no disturbing changes in breathing from variations in depths of unconsciousness. Its administration is simple, too.

A slender, flexible needle of silver or gold alloy is slipped skillfully into the space around the great nerve trunks of the spinal cord running down from the brain to the trunk and extremities. A single dose of the anesthetic agent can be injected through the needle or a rubber tube can be connected to it and the patient turned on his back, leaving the needle in place. Here the anesthetist can control the amount and level of anesthesia, injecting more of the drug until the level of loss of sensation creeps upward, stopping when it is exactly high enough for the job at hand, replenishing the supply from time to time so the sensation will not return until the operation is completed. This continuous spinal anesthesia is ideal for long reconstructions upon the extremities, plastic skin grafts to burned legs, bone grafts to replace the blasting effect of shrapnel and high-powered projectiles—in fact, any operation below the middle of the trunk.

Or again anesthetists may use the new caudal injection, which has proved such a boon to women in childbirth, inserting a needle into the tiny foramen at the base of the spine, injecting a small amount of solution from time to time, and thus carrying on the pain relief for hours. All these are variations of the subscience of regional anesthesia, the vast field of pain relief opened up to surgeons by the discovery of novocain and its derivatives.

It is easy to understand how the dentist, thrusting his needle deep into the tissues inside the mouth, can, with a single injection of novocain, block off the nerve supplying sensation to all the teeth of one side of the jaw. No more imagination is required to understand how a long needle, thrust by skillful hands across the middle of the collar bone and deep into the tissues of the neck, can seek out and find there the great nerve trunks of the brachial plexus of the arm and block out all sensation by an injection of the anesthetic fluid around these pathways. A needle inserted into the muscles beside the lower rim of a broken rib can in a second remove all pain, or if several ribs are blocked simultaneously, allow a window to be made into the chest to drain an accumulation of pus from a retained piece of shrapnel.

Ever since the first explorer went into the South American jungles years ago, tall tales have been drifting out concerning the poisons used on the Indian arrows, poisons that could kill an animal or a man in a matter of seconds by widespread paralysis. Modern pharmacologic science identified the poison as a form of curare, a vegetable product of certain plants with the power of breaking the flow of nerve impulses to the voluntary muscles and thus achieving complete muscular relaxation, often a valuable aid in major surgery.

Although some investigators still feel that even the highly purified curare derivatives and curarelike drugs now in use are too powerful and too dangerous for routine anesthesia, conservative anesthetists stoutly maintain their value when properly controlled. Given as a continuous injection, coupled with Pentothal Sodium and nitrous-oxide anesthesia and rigidly controlled, curare seems an important adjunct that will continue to be used in specific cases that demand its relaxing properties.

Another agent favored by many anesthetists is a dilute solution of novocain given intravenously, an unheard-of thing twenty years ago, proving that one man's poison may be another's meat—if he knows how to eat it. Even more startling is hypotensive anesthesia, used in operations in which considerable bleeding is expected. Here a drug called trimethaphan camphorsulfonate is used to reduce the blood pressure to a very low level during the operation and thus avoid what might be an otherwise fatal hemorrhage.

Two specters have haunted anesthetists and surgeons since

time immemorial. One is shock developing during major surgery. Modern anesthetic practice seeks to prevent this by blood transfusions and the injection of plasma or plasma substitutes at the first sign of falling blood pressure, or even before. When shock does develop, however, in spite of these precautions, an adrenal-cortex hormone called F-cortisone is often lifesaving, as are newer forms of epinephrine, a product of the pharmacology laboratories that has far more powerful artery-constricting effects than the old, familiar adrenalin of long ago.

Still another indication for cortisone treatment is in patients who have been taking the drug for other reasons. Sudden death under anesthesia in such cases is not unheard of, presumably because the adrenal gland has become atrophied or lazy while not required to supply its own hormone. Treatment with cortisone prior to operation will usually prevent this unhappy complication.

The other great surgical specter is cardiac arrest, cessation of the heartbeat during operation from no discernible cause. One of the greatest advances of modern surgical science—described in the chapter on anesthesia only because it happens most frequently during operations—is the technique, now in wide use, of restarting the heartbeat in such cases. Treating this emergency requires split-second action, but fortunately an operating team is usually already functioning when it occurs. The chest must be opened as quickly as possible, ignoring surgical cleanliness if necessary, to expose the heart.

Stopping of the heartbeat during operation is of two forms, a simple cessation of motion and a condition called fibrillation. In fibrillation, the muscle of the heart ventricle writhes in an aimless motion that completely defeats its purpose of pumping blood. The first condition, simple cessation of motion, is treated by massage, kneading the heart with the hand until it takes up its normal rhythm. The second is handled preferably by applying a de-fibrillator, a device that shoots several jolts of electricity directly into the heart, stopping the aimless fibrillation. Following this, massage will usually restore the normal beat.

It was this condition of fibrillation that stopped the heart of the woman mentioned in the opening paragraph of this book, and exactly the technique described above started it again, fifty minutes later. Meanwhile the patient was without pulse or respiration, except that induced by those seeking to save her. This is about as near death as anyone can come, and still live.

Her own opinion? "I am sure that I was dead for fifty minutes."

Control of shock; control of pain; and next, control of infection, and a signal victory in the war against man's relentless microbe enemies.

4.

GOD'S POWDERS

Penicillin—Its discovery by Dr. Fleming—Why it was not developed or used for many years—Sulfanilamide—Uses in connection with surgery—Its limitations—Sulfapyridine—Sulfathiazole—Sulfadiazine—Penicillin, isolating and producing it for wide use—What it does—New antibiotics—The "-mycins"

History, Providence, Fate—call it what you will—seems to have a habit of fitting the man to the needs of humanity. How else explain the sequence of events that placed Pasteur in his laboratory when a chicken cholera virus, partially attenuated by accident, failed to kill the fowl into which it was injected, thereby revealing at a later date the intricate reaction of antibody formation that we call immunity? How else explain the trail of fire set up in the brain of obstetrician Semmelweis when he first realized that the death of his friend Kolletschka from a needle prick during an autopsy resulted from the same infection as that causing the child-bed fever killing mothers contaminated by the unwashed hands of their *accoucheurs?*

In 1929 another such coincidence of medical scientist and miracle took place, unheralded, leaving the world for more than ten years completely unaware that there had been isolated a drug that was the greatest microbe hunter of them all, a drug that cured fatal diseases overnight with no more disturbance than the four-hourly pain of a needle prick.

Like Pasteur, like Semmelweis, like all the hundreds of medical pioneers who have given us lifesaving discoveries, mild Dr. Alexander Fleming, puttering about among his cultures in St. Mary's Hospital of the University of London, was merely the agent waiting—unwittingly, no doubt—to culminate a series of discoveries forming the bricks from which the final structure was built.

Who knows how far back go the basic discoveries that gave us penicillin, the master miracle drug of all time? Perhaps it was to Pasteur and Joubert in 1877, noting—as good scientists note every occurrence, no matter how unimportant—that certain air-borne microbes inhibited the growth of fatal anthrax bacilli. Perhaps it was to D'Herelle, who first saw the germ-destroying properties of the microbe-that-preys-on-microbes, bacteriophage.

Whatever the source, the important thing is that on a day in 1929, Dr. Alexander Fleming was investigating peculiarities in the growth of an ordinary laboratory microbe, the staphylococcus, which grew on almost any kind of medium as discrete, whitish plaques. After treatment with the Gram stain, they looked under the microscope like grapes, clusters of brilliant purple organisms. It was almost omnipresent, this staphylococcus, causing such innocuous things as pimples and boils, and many times less innocuous carbuncles. Sometimes it ran unchecked through the body, with no known agent to curb its wildfire spread.

But it wasn't the death-causing properties of the staphylococcus—or "staph," as doctors learned to call it in their studies—that Dr. Fleming was investigating. His was an ordinary study of mutations in colonies, and it called for frequently opening the petri dishes—flat glass plates in which bacteria are grown in the laboratory—to study the size and shape of the colonies under the microscope. Inevitably, many plates became contaminated—sometimes from the bacteria that float everywhere in the air, sometimes from the mold spores that, as every housewife knows, need only the combination of bread, time, and moisture to produce a wrinkled green covering that makes food inedible.

But why should one particular plate become contaminated with a peculiar sort of mold with the rhythmic name of *penicillium notatum?* And a mold that had been found in, of all places, decaying hyssop in Norway.

Other molds had contaminated other plates, resulting only in the discarding of the particular culture. How easy it would have been for this particular contamination, too, to have been tossed into the bucket to which discarded cultures were consigned. But Dr. Fleming was a scientist, and he didn't discard cultures without looking at them just because the last hundred, or the last thousand, had been harmless air molds. He studied this plate, and what he saw made history. Not right then, but it set in motion the chain of events that has resulted in countless lives saved on the battlefield, innumerable children released from the doom of pneumococcus meningitis. And—this may be its greatest contribution—the eradication of a great scourge from the world, the killer that has only recently been brought from behind the screen of hypocrisy and false prudery that has hidden progress in its control and exposed for the murderer that it is—syphilis.

What Dr. Fleming saw was no startling change; in fact, he was the first to admit that probably many others had seen it before him. But the right combination of staph colonies, plus penicillium notatum, plus a mind that thought in terms of germ killing by antibiotic substances had never before occurred. Dr. Fleming himself modestly put it:

"I was always on the lookout for new bacterial inhibitors, and when I noticed on a culture plate that the staphylococcus colonies in the neighborhood of a mold had faded away, I was sufficiently interested in the antibacterial substance produced by the mold to pursue the subject."

Realizing that this particular mold had a property that other molds did not possess, he went ahead to obtain a pure culture of penicillium notatum which had gobbled up the staph cultures in its neighborhood. He grew this powerful invader in special broths and identified it. Then he carried the study even further; he tried the effect of this broth from a penicillium culture on colonies of other bacteria, with remarkable results.

Against many common laboratory germs, the kind that occur in diseases every day, this new antibacterial substance produced by the mold growth was remarkably lethal, in fact *two or three times as strong as pure carbolic acid!*

When injected into rats, to test for the bad effects it might have on humans, it was found to be amazingly well tolerated.

Only in a few instances was there any reaction, and subsequent purification of the active principle has shown that these were more from by-products having no significance in medicine and now completely eliminated from commercial penicillin.

The therapeutic uses of penicillin were not immediately evident for a number of reasons. One of the greatest was the relative instability of the substance produced by the mold. It was soluble in water, a great help, but its strength diminished rapidly in a few days, if allowed to stand at room temperature. Only neutral solutions seemed relatively stable and these were killed by heating, such as is used to sterilize ordinary ampules of drugs.

Dr. Fleming himself recognized the potentialities of the substance—especially when it was demonstrated that it was markedly nontoxic to test rats—and suggested that it might be of great value in surface infections with staphylococcus, streptococcus, and the other germs against which it was effective. It was even used in the laboratory for culturing the elusive influenza bacillus, which is usually smothered by growths from other germs when sputum or cough cultures are made. Penicillin allowed the influenza germ to grow unchecked, but killed most of the others instantly.

Penicillin continued as little more than a laboratory curiosity, although in 1931 Dr. Fleming said: "It is quite likely that it, or a chemical of a similar nature, will be used in the treatment of septic wounds." The substance was there, the method of its growth was known; it remained for chemists and other research workers to evolve a method by which the pure agent could be isolated and prepared in a manner permitting its use in medicine.

Meanwhile events occurred that obscured for several years any further development of this powerful mold substance. In 1933 German chemist Gerhard Domagk and a co-worker published their report that a strange new compound they had been working on was a miraculously effective protection for mice against fatal inoculation with streptococcus. It was just a laboratory observation, and it is probable that at first its discoverers had no idea what a powerful weapon they had discovered in man's fight for existence and health. Only several years later did there appear on world markets a reddish-brown substance that quickly demonstrated its power to kill many germs.

Doctors recognized at once that in this new drug they had a razor-edged weapon against swift-spreading germ invasion, which often left them completely helpless before its onslaught. And recognizing its value, they sought to know more about it. Chemists began to study this new product of the mother substance of so many drugs, coal tar, to analyze its structure and seek to derive from it new and perhaps more effective compounds.

Meanwhile other workers were studying the effect of the drug when administered in various ways. If sulfanilamide was so powerful when swallowed as a tablet, they reasoned, why not concentrate the fire at the place where it would do the most good, the infected area itself. It was a reasonable idea, and so doctors began treating wounds with sulfanilamide, sprinkling it into lacerations, washing out cavities with irrigating solutions, even injecting it into abdomens inflamed by peritonitis. Medical literature blossomed out with hundreds of reports of cases in which surgeons had poured sulfanilamide into compound fractures, into infected wounds, wherever it seemed that bacteria needed to be attacked. They also gave the drug by mouth and by injection, and no one could be quite certain where the credit lay.

There was no doubt that credit was due. Infection rates in compound fractures and in all sorts of contaminated wounds dropped. Wounds healed without pus, fractures without the bone-destroying infection of osteomyelitis. Doctors began to look upon the sulfa drugs—for other and far more effective ones were being made by the chemists, first sulfapyridine, then sulfathiazole, and sulfadiazine—as cure-alls. People even referred to them jokingly as God's Powders.

Conflicting reports began to pour in, too. Some hard-headed surgeons said the results weren't entirely attributable to the local use of the new drugs, that wounds would heal if you cleansed them thoroughly. Most important of all, however, they gave the drugs by mouth or by injection, building up a concentration in the blood stream. They even quoted figures that seemed to prove that local use was not of much value.

Then came Pearl Harbor. Overnight catastrophe struck and hundreds of wounded poured into the hospitals in Honolulu and elsewhere on the Hawaiian Islands. Trained surgeons were waiting, blood plasma, transfusions, even a trick instrument for locating foreign bodies that turned out to be not a trick at all but a valuable help in what was usually a very difficult job. And too, there were packages of sulfanilamide powder to be sifted into the wounds, hundreds of tablets of the sulfa drugs to be taken by mouth.

The results were history, a triumph for modern surgery, and a preview of the results in lifesaving that enabled the Medical Corps of the armed forces to save more than ninety-six out of every hundred wounded who reached a hospital.

And so there was a rush to use sulfanilamide in all wounds. It had done wonders at Pearl Harbor; why keep it from anyone? Why try to accumulate figures? What difference did it make anyway, so long as infection was prevented? What difference, indeed, except that doctors are scientists and scientists are devoted to the truth? What difference except that if the good effects were not entirely from dumping the powder into the wounds, some doctors might get a false sense of confidence in local use of the drug and let up on internal use of it, might not even insist that wounded men or injured civilians keep on taking the drugs internally.

A few hard-headed doctors went on checking results, such things as whether dumping a lot of powdered drug into a wound didn't interfere with healing, didn't increase the incidence of wound disruption. They were voices crying in the wilderness, those hard-headed investigators, and often they were laughed at, even castigated verbally for their pains, their conservatism in not jumping on the bandwagon that kept playing the tune that local sulfonamide was a cure-all. Thanks to those few who stuck it out, we know a great deal more now than we did before the war.

But while the hue and cry was developing over the local use of sulfanilamide in wounds, chemists and physicians were working together to discover new uses for these miracle drugs. Sulfanilamide was wonderful, everyone agreed on that, but it was also a little disappointing. Pneumonia still took nearly one in every four who contracted it, in spite of serum and oxygen therapy. Now if sulfanilamide would only destroy the elongated, dark-staining bugs of pneumonia, the pneumococci, that would be a wonderful thing.

But it didn't destroy pneumonia germs. Give the drug until the patients were a deep-blue color, until they vomited, had headaches, and sometimes even developed the dangerous destructive disease of the white blood cells that sometimes followed administration of the drug that doctors knew as "agranulocytosis"—nothing happened.

Then word came from England of a new compound, a chemical that knocked the pneumococcus cold. Identified as a sulfanilamide derivative, sulfapyridine soon demonstrated its power to destroy the pneumonia germ. Given to a patient with a lung half solid from the exudates of the pneumococcus infection, with rising fever and incontrovertible evidence of a severe pneumonia, with more than one chance in four of not coming through at all—a miraculous thing occurred. The temperature dropped often in a matter of hours, toxicity disappeared, and the patient started feeling better right away.

The X-ray showed that the patient still had the consolidation of pneumonia in his chest; its disappearance was expedited little if any over the normal time, but the patient showed little evidence of its presence. It was difficult even to keep him in bed the required time. For patients unable to take it by mouth, the drug could be injected directly into the veins, stopping the pneumonia germs as effectively as a bazooka stopped a tank head-on. Here was a miracle indeed; in one winter, pneumonia was conquered.

But sulfapyridine, too, was not the cure-all. There were still a lot of germs it didn't entirely kill. For instance, neither sulfanilamide nor sulfapyridine could even dent the staphylococcus, the grapelike clusters of violet-colored germs that cause painful carbuncles, dangerous kidney abscesses, frequently fatal blood-stream infections. And too, both sulfanilamide and sulfapyridine tended to make the patient sick, both upset stomachs, both caused a certain percentage of unpleasant effects on the white blood cells and an often troublesome anemia. Something was needed to overcome these effects.

That, too, was not long in coming. Chemists discovered a

new sulfanilamide derivative. This one they called sulfathiazole, and now they had a really big gun to add to their artillery against disease. Sulfathiazole did everything sulfanilamide had done, everything sulfapyridine had done, did them more effectively and with fewer side effects, and in addition was certain death for many other bacteria—the staphylococcus, the gonococcus, the meningococcus. The list grew all the time.

Now here was a white crystalline substance that could really be labeled God's Powder. Not only did it work internally, but it seemed to work externally, too, in wounds, in the peritoneum. It was not as soluble as sulfanilamide in wounds—that was a drawback—but it was absorbed more slowly and the effect locally, if there really was an effect, was much more prolonged.

Sulfathiazole enjoyed a year of popularity before its near twin brother came along, sulfadiazine. Here was another germ fighter extraordinary, the culmination of chemical and medical research since sulfanilamide first turned up as a streptococcus destroyer in the bodies of mice in 1933. For sulfadiazine was the least toxic of all the sulfa drugs, and the most effective.

We had come a long way since 1933, and many lives had been saved. Meanwhile, in the rush to use the miracle drugs derived from coal tar, penicillin had still remained little more than a laboratory curiosity. Some work had been done on it, enough to show that it could be used in abscess cavities, and could even be purified to a point where it could be injected into the body, often with miraculous results. But it was still hard to make it in more than very minute quantities, certainly not enough for the extensive experimental studies that should be made if its true value was to be revealed.

Dr. E. Chain and Dr. H. W. Florey, of Oxford, had been working patiently for years at the Sir William Dunn School of Pathology, seeking to isolate some of the many antibiotic agents—the name given to substances produced by one microbe that inhibited or destroyed the growth of others—of which penicillin is only one. They studied pyocyanase, a substance produced by the musty-smelling germ of green pus, which Otto Loew and others had recognized and attempted to use medically as early as 1899. They knew about Dr. Fleming's work, they knew how unstable penicillin had proved to be, but they also knew that under certain conditions the activity of penicillin could be demonstrated in the broth from which a culture had been grown for a number of weeks. This encouraging fact, coupled with the known range of activity of penicillin, seemed to make investigation into its chemical structure and methods of isolation well worth while.

Dr. Chain and Dr. Florey found a number of things, all interesting to the chemist and the bacteriologist, many interesting to the casual reader. In the first place penicillin is a very weak acid, liable to chemical disintegration as such acids often are. But combined with other substances to form salts, particularly sodium and calcium, penicillin becomes much more stable. Now it seemed that Chain and Florey were on the right track. When they found that the culture broth on which the mold is grown—the mother substance from which penicillin itself is obtained—can be extracted with ether and then shaken with an alkali to form stable salts, they knew they were on the trail of a real discovery. From there on methods of purification become more and more complicated as more and more nearly pure solutions are obtained.

What is this miracle drug like? In the laboratory it is a green, felted mass, floating in a bottle on top of a broth that looks like concentrated bouillon. As the mold grows, the penicillin is dissolved in the broth on which the mass floats and it is from this that the active principle is isolated.

Without the speeded-up research that accompanied wartime activities it is doubtful if penicillin would have been nearly as available as it is now for many, many years. However, as a result of the research of Dr. Chain and Dr. Florey, American scientists were able to work out a method of growing the mold in very large vats, feeding it on corn steep liquor, a product of corn that served as an extremely valuable culture medium. In this way large-scale production of penicillin was made possible very quickly, accounting for the fact that so much of it was available for use during World War II. Progress in penicillin production has, of course, continued since the war and now it is widely available and used almost as regularly as aspirin.

Unfortunately, penicillin is not a cure-all. A whole host of mankind's microbe enemies are not affected by it, particularly the viruses which cause many serious illnesses. Too, the widespread use of penicillin in every conceivable type of illness, from the common cold to athlete's foot, has caused many people to develop a sensitivity to it that makes later injection dangerous. More and more patients are developing severe skin eruptions from it, a form of allergic reaction, and occasionally a death results. It is still by far the most widely used of the antibiotic drugs, but more and more doctors are inclined to be cautious when no definite indication for treatment with penicillin exists.

In one field, the treatment of venereal disease, penicillin is without a peer. Take for example gonorrhea, the scourge that raged through the ranks of men and women unchecked until the advent of the sulfa drugs, and in many cases was not cured by them. This little-talked-of disease caused much loss of time from work in industry and in the armed services —where, to the surprise of most people, its occurrence was much less frequent than in civil life. In addition, many young women's reproductive functions were forever destroyed by this infection which, acquired innocently or not, had the same ultimate result.

The results of penicillin treatment in gonorrhea astonished even the most sanguine of therapists. A few dollars' worth of the drug usually cures completely a fresh case of gonorrhea. Complications require only a little more. Only in exceptional instances does the treatment fail, and then larger doses usually effect a cure.

New methods of preparing penicillin have made it cheaper, and many state health departments now give the drug free for the treatment of indigent cases of venereal disease. No one will quarrel with the statement that penicillin has truly revolutionized the treatment of one of our greatest scourges.

Dwarfing even the results obtained with gonorrhea, however, are those obtained with syphilis, a disease so widespread that it has been estimated that one out of every ten—in many places a much higher proportion—of the population carries the deadly corkscrew germs in his blood.

Consider what syphilis meant only a few years ago: weekly injections of arsenical drugs, supplemented by bismuth, for a year, or perhaps more. An expense in cost of drugs alone, enormous, in loss of time throughout the country, incalculable; in hospital beds devoted to treating brains diseased by syphilis, staggering. A moral and emotional drain on the country greater than almost any other of its kind, greater even than much publicized tuberculosis.

What can penicillin offer to one whose blood gives the positive reaction of the Kahn and Wasserman tests of syphilis, whose tissues teem with the spirochete? Nothing less than a cure more certain than even Dr. Paul Ehrlich dreamed of, as he injected compound after compound in his attempt to find the one best suited to tackle the spirochete of syphilis, stopping only when the six hundred and sixth drug combination turned out to be what he was seeking. One week of penicillin is equivalent to a year or more of arsenic treatment, preventing thousands of dollars of expense, thousands of cases of insanity, and hordes of children who would have been born when they had better died in the womb, with congenital or inherited syphilis.

Nor is penicillin the only one of the antibiotic substances that aids man against disease. Many others, some miraculously effective, have resulted from the speeded-up research of the first decade since war's end.

Some twenty-nine years ago, Dr. Selman A. Waksman, of Rutgers University, began to study soil cultures, particularly the molds found in dirt. From his studies have come a whole new field of antibiotic science, that of literally saving lives with dirt.

From a mold cultured outside Dr. Waksman's laboratory window came streptomycin, a powerful germ fighter attacking many bacteria not affected by penicillin at all. Scientists in the laboratories of Parke, Davis and Company discovered a still newer agent in soil, a mold from which came potent chloromycetin, which has also been synthesized chemically. Workers at the Lederle Laboratories developed a powerful yellow germ fighter called Aureomycin, while a second group isolated another weapon in Terramycin.

As new antibiotics roll from the laboratory production line, each touted as more powerful than the preceding ones, even the physician is sometimes bewildered and wonders if the day is not far off when the man-microbe war will be won completely, with no germs left to cause disease. At this writing, such a happy consequence does not seem likely, however. For as insects become resistant to DDT, so germs develop an immunity to various antibiotic drugs. Particularly is this true of the staphylococcus, which ordinarily causes no great trouble, but when other bacteria are destroyed by the drugs, may become the causative agent in severe and sometimes fatal illness. Fortunately, each year brings a new weapon with an even greater promise of eventual conquest of the ubiquitous microbe.

At the outbreak of World War II, however, penicillin was still a laboratory curiosity and the other antibiotic agents had not been discovered. Even so, shock was well on the way to being conquered and discoveries in the field of anesthesia, including the new injected sleep, already hailed a new era of surgery. And war surgery itself had been tested and tried in another strange laboratory, the Laboratory for War.

∨

5.

LABORATORY FOR WAR

Surgery in World War II—96 per cent of wounded saved—Surgery in previous wars—Dr. Winnet Orr—Dr. Trueta in the Spanish Civil War—Gas gangrene—Taking surgery to the front—Welch bacillus in wounds—Closed plaster treatment—Applications of war to peacetime surgery

Modern wars are no longer won on the battlefield; they are won in the laboratory. World War II made this fact abundantly clear, for it was a succession of scientific discoveries, culminating in the atomic bomb, that finally brought the enemy to his knees. Less well known but equally true is the fact that the success of doctors in saving more than 96 per cent of the wounded who reached hospitals was also the product of research in many laboratories—but most of all a new "Laboratory for War" during the late nineteen thirties, the Spanish Civil War.

It didn't all begin in Spain. It actually began a long time before, perhaps as far back as the sixteenth century, when Ambroise Paré noticed that wounds so dirty as to be teeming with maggots were often clean and healthy. This discovery was later effectively applied by Dr. William S. Baer, the famed orthopedist of Johns Hopkins; he found the cleaning agent to be allantoin, the strange tissue-dissolving substance secreted by maggots.

Perhaps the whole story began with Dominique Jean Larrey, another Frenchman, who was surgeon to one of the armies of Napoleon; his ambulances took an active part in the

battle of Austerlitz, and his skill as a surgeon was so great
that he could perform the most formidable operations in
minutes—without anesthesia.

Or it may have begun with Ignaz Semmelweis, the Magyar
with the funny name, who discovered how the streptococcus
of childbed fever is transmitted to the lining of the mother's
womb—certainly a great bleeding wound as a result of recently being bereft of its embryonic occupant—by the hands
of the surgeon who attended her in her hour of travail; Semmelweis, who died insane from pounding his head against
the wall of entrenched medical ignorance and stupidity. Certainly it was not so recent as either Pasteur or Lister, with
their theories of antiseptic surgery that were to revolutionize
the practice of their ancient art.

With all the accumulated wealth of medical knowledge,
the world should have been ready for the great holocaust of
1914, but medical history shows that such was not the case.
Scientific progress, like that in other fields, does not move
in a straight and rising line. Rather it moves crabwise, by
alternate rushes and retreats. World War I caught medical
science in one of those periods of retreat, when not even the
wise principles of Ambroise Paré—that wounds should be enlarged to let out infection, to remove foreign bodies in the
form of clothing, missiles, and bits of bone and dead tissue—
were adhered to.

Military surgery was in a state of therapeutic nihilism
when World War I began; it had no methods tried and
found good in the laboratory of war as it did in World War
II. Instead, a let-alone principle was adhered to at first, with
disastrous results. Infection flamed through the bodies of
nearly all who fell in the first battles of that early war.
Mortality rose, until a bullet through the belly was as good
as a death warrant. A bullet through the thigh often resulted
in gas gangrene, with the loss of the injured member as the
most optimistic prognosis.

Then, with the effects of their tragic neglect filling the
hospitals, European surgeons realized that infection is an
inevitable accompaniment of war wounds. They sought to
prevent infection, and the French invented the ingenious
idea of trying to remove the wound, cutting away damaged

skin, muscle, even bone, slashing restraining fascial barriers, ingeniously slipping deep into the wounds rubber tubes, through which they squirted every few hours the magic Carrel-Dakin solution, which was to kill all remaining bacteria.

It did good work, too, that bleaching-powder solution smelling of chlorine. It cleaned up infection and allowed wounds to heal. But it could not accomplish miracles, could not attack infection already deeply seated in the body during the long hours, even days, of evacuation to the first hospital far back of the line of battle.

And so the process of evolution moved forward, continually forward this time. The British began to operate on seriously wounded patients as far forward as their field ambulances, well back of the front line itself yet far closer to it than any hospital had ever been before. The Americans, too, were adopting some such system, taking surgery to the patient, cutting the time lag that determined success or failure in treating the dangerously wounded soldier.

World War I ended in its very infancy compared with the modern struggle for survival, through which we have only recently passed, and there were to be no more wars after that—so they said. Surgeons over the world were laying some of the groundwork in traumatic surgery, increasingly more important as America became more and more industrialized.

A few men, especially Dr. Winnet Orr, American orthopedist, had a vision of what might have been common knowledge had the European war lasted a few years longer. Dr. Orr operated on wounds, more specifically compound fractures, and enclosed them in plaster casts, adopting the until then unheard of practice of sealing off the entire wound by putting plaster directly over it. Secretions accumulated, the smell soon became almost unbearable, but those wounded soldiers journeyed across the Atlantic with their casts unchanged and arrived here in good condition. From this work came the Orr treatment of osteomyelitis, infection of the bone, which was well on the way to becoming standard over the world before the sulfonamide drugs cut down the incidence of bone destruction in that dramatic disease, as it did the ravages of so many other infections.

The principles were ready, clearly delineated, for another

conflict. It required only a little smoothing over, a little knocking off of the rough edges, to put them into practice. When Hitler used the civil war in Spain as a laboratory, he set the stage for those finishing touches. The first casualties coming under the marvelously skillful hands of Dr. J. Trueta in the General Hospital of Catalonia began the experiment. Rather it should be said that it was not even then in the experimental stage.

Trueta says himself in his book, *Treatment of War Wounds and Fractures,* that he had applied his methods to industrial accidents but his reports of outstanding success had been received with the skepticism common to medical men presented with something so radically new and different from any of the older methods of treatment that they are for the moment unable to comprehend its ramifications.

Trueta's methods rapidly became standard throughout the Republican Army, and results were immediately dramatic. Gas gangrene fell to a trifling percentage, almost negligible when compared with its ravages during World War I with the then standard treatment of *débridement* and irrigation. Streptococcic infection, the bane of the war surgeon, yielded almost completely.

These were not entirely the results of Trueta's methods, for at the same time forward-looking surgeons of the Spanish Republican Army, headed by the Chief Surgical Consultant, Colonel J. H. d'Harcourt, had added another dramatic note to this symphony of saving lives. More than ever before, more than even the British, who had had the daring to operate on abdominal wounds at field ambulance stations in World War I, the Spanish doctors in uniform were taking surgery to the patient. They did this through an ingenious system of hospitals and ambulance evacuation lines, described by Major Douglas W. Jolly in his fascinating account of the workings of the medical service in Spain, *Field Surgery in Total War.*

Briefly, this new method consisted of three essential elements. First was a Casualty Classification Post, corresponding approximately to the second echelon in the system used by the American Army, the Collecting Station. Here trained officers carried out a work that on the face of it might not seem important but that actually determined the success of the entire system. As the cases came through, they separated those in which the time lag meant success or failure. These they labeled cases of "First Urgency," and shot quickly a little way to a small portable hospital set up in a protected spot, often an old wine cellar, a cave, or even an abandoned railway tunnel.

Complete in every detail, limited only in size, this hospital always had available a surgeon whose skill and experience fitted him to handle any wound that came his way. Here for the first time it was possible to do an almost unheard of thing, operate on wounds in a matter of hours after they occurred—always less than five or six, for that was considered the deadline of infection. Here abdominal wounds could be operated on before uncontrollable peritonitis had set in, sucking wounds of the chest could be closed, and brain wounds cleaned up and prepared for evacuation back to the Special Base Hospitals, where corps of specialists waited to handle just such delicate problems.

Consider the work of these hospitals and it immediately becomes apparent why classification was such an important function. Jam up these little hospitals of "First Urgency" with wounded who could safely be evacuated farther back to the Number Two Hospital and a lot of seriously wounded would have to wait, wait when every moment meant that the bacteria in their untreated wounds were attacking body tissues, consolidating positions from which they could be rooted out only by prolonged and painful treatment, if at all. No wonder the Spanish surgeons agreed that the doctor in the Classification Post was the key man.

There was one weakness about these Number One Hospitals, a weakness that no one has yet been able to correct, except, perhaps, by having the hospital right beside an emergency airfield, from which patients could be evacuated quickly and safely. Once an abdominal case was operated on—less important in a compound fracture but still important, and absolutely important in a brain case—the patient must not be moved for at least a week. That meant the hospitals had to stay put, or if they moved, went forward, they had to leave personnel to care for those bedded by the operation.

In a forward-moving operation this was all very well, and

sometimes the system, elastic as it was, worked beautifully by having the hospitals follow the troops, leapfrogging the Number Two Hospital over the Number One to become the new Number One. But reverses meant capture, and the civilized rules of Geneva did not always have much weight. It was a weakness of the system, but the advantages far exceeded the drawbacks.

Let us see for a moment, before going on to the application of the discoveries of the medical Laboratory for War, just what was accomplished by Trueta and the other gallant medical soldiers of Spain and their volunteer allies. A few brief statistics tell the story more graphically than any words. In one series of cases reported by d'Harcourt and others in the *British Medical Journal*, out of 5,000 major fracture cases, many of them the dangerous compound breaks, there were only thirty-seven deaths. A mortality of less than three-quarters of one per cent!

Never in the history of medicine and surgery had such a vast experiment been conducted in saving human lives. Never had such results been obtained in preventing gas gangrene, the "death that stalks the battlefield." Such results are not always obtainable, for not always is it possible to get the right combination of early and adequate surgery. But working on these principles proved feasible in the Spanish laboratory, and American, British, and Russian surgeons went on to work out the system of care of the wounded pointed out by Trueta and his associates, which gave such wonderful results in the infinitely larger-scaled campaigns of World War II.

Military surgeons are faced with a difficult problem, wherever they work. All war wounds sustained on the battlefield are infected. Often these wounds contain one particular germ, a vitriolic sort of fat little bacillus that sometimes doubles itself up into a small round ball that the bacteriologists call a spore. It is practically impossible to destroy by heat, by antisepsis, or by any of the accepted methods of germ killing. This fat germ has been known to doctors for many years, ever since beloved pathologist "Popsie" Welch of Johns Hopkins, first established its identity—established it, so the story goes, from the remains of a corpse that disrupted its own funeral by exploding. Since then it has been known over the world as the Welch bacillus, or simply the bacillus of gas gangrene.

Now, this Welch bacillus and the equally malignant group of which it is a member, known as the clostridia, have two peculiar characteristics. One is that, unlike most living things, they do not require oxygen for their growth; in fact, they seem to thrive better where it is not present in high concentrations. The other is that they produce poisons far deadlier than that of the king cobra, poisons that can kill a man in a matter of hours.

Anaerobes, as the air-haters are called, are normally present in the excreta of animals, which means that troops fighting over highly cultivated farming country, such as much of Europe, are frequently subject to contamination of wounds by anaerobes. Even in the desert, in wide spaces that are relatively uninhabited, the British found that approximately 30 per cent of wounds were contaminated by the malignant gas-gangrene microbes.

But it wasn't always necessary for cultivated soil to get into wounds to infect them with the gas bacillus. The British carried on an elaborate series of studies in Egypt and Libya to discover if there were any other sources of infection. And they found, interestingly enough, that the Tommies carried with them the source of their infections—their uniforms.

British medical officers went about snipping portions of soldiers' uniforms and cultivating them for the dread gas organisms. They took twenty-five "battle dresses" and found the malignant bacteria in six tunics and eleven trousers, which fitted in with the observation common to all medical officers who have handled the wounded that leg wounds are always worse than arm wounds as far as gas gangrene is concerned. They even cultured the abbreviated khaki drill used for summer wear and found much the same thing. Small wonder, then, that about one out of every three wounds was contaminated with the gas-gangrene bacillus.

But contamination doesn't mean infection, fortunately for those unlucky enough to be wounded. There are several stages the bacteria may go through before actually invading the body. And they may be stopped in any of the stages. The British knew how to stop them, as witness the fact that only about one per cent of those actually contaminated with the clostridia developed what could actually be termed gas gangrene. And as they knew what gas gangrene was, it was not a question of those British surgeons being unable to recognize it.

The picture had lingered in the minds of all those surgeons who worked in World War I, lingered as perhaps their most vivid and horrible memory of all they had seen in battle. For real gas gangrene is a horrible thing. Deep in a thigh wound the germs find all the conditions favorable for their growth. Muscle tissue, torn, lacerated, perhaps burned from the heat of a screaming fragment of shrapnel—that is the first prerequisite. Damaged blood supply to muscles, bones, tissues, is another. A small wound, hiding from the inexpert observer the extent of the deeper injury and leading him into a false sense of security that may not let him treat that small wound as ruthlessly as he would a larger, gaping one, is still another.

Given these three prerequisites, gas gangrene is an almost certain conclusion, sulfonamides or no sulfonamides, serum or no serum, even when penicillin is also used. Here, deep in the tissues, almost completely bereft of oxygen, the fat little germs grow fatter, bisect themselves in the process of reproduction, and double their number time and time again until they invade the tissues, producing gas that opens up tissue planes between muscles, nerves, and blood vessels, clearing a fresh path along which this germ invasion can move rapidly toward the more vital portions of the body.

And with all this, the toxins are pouring from those busy little germs, poisons of a potency almost unbelievable. In a matter of hours the stricken soldier begins to mutter with delirium. The injured leg throbs, and he screams with pain that is almost unbearable in its throbbing intensity. The limb swells under the very eyes of the surgeons, swells and grows tense with gas that crackles beneath the pressing finger.

Sometimes, but not often enough to be an infallible sign, there is even a characteristic smell. Some have called it a "mortuary smell," certainly an appropriate odor, for fully one out of three who come to this stage finds his way to the impersonal slabs of the deadhouse. Even the skin takes on a suggestive color. Frequently it is white, the dead-white pallor of marble. Or sometimes it is bronze, the deeper brownish color of a bronze casket. Gas gangrene is not misnamed as the "death that stalks the battlefield."

But strangely enough in those cases reported from the Spanish war, the ones treated by Trueta's tradition-breaking closed-plaster treatment, death had not stalked the battlefield. In fact, gas gangrene had been a rare occurrence, even without the protection of "God's Powders," which weren't even in use at that time.

What, then, had been done to these men that was so different from the treatment of World War I? Was it the plaster casts? Evidently not, for patients had been put in plaster in this war and had developed gas gangrene.

Was it because the treatment had not been radical enough in World War I, once a wounded soldier was found to have the germs of gas gangrene in his body? Certainly not, for amputation had been the rule. Many limbs were sacrificed because a little gas developed in the tissues of the thigh, a little foul, thin pus escaped from the wound, a little fever indicated some absorption of toxins. It was evident to all military surgeons that more must be learned about this dread enemy of both attacker and attacked in war time.

And so the British medical officers started working on this problem. They had the material to study, for they were at war. A great battle was surging back and forth across the shores of the Mediterranean, sometimes in thickly settled towns and farming lands, ideal sources of clostridia, sometimes in sandy deserts, where there would be few if any of the germs of gas gangrene. They investigated every case, they cultured the various members of the clostridia family, including the most frequent invader, the Welch bacillus. They read the medical officers' descriptions of those who died and those who lived. They checked back on the original operative records describing the treatment of the original wounds. And they found many interesting things, things that enabled our country, coming late into the war, to keep down the incidence of gas gangrene in our own troops.

The main thing those British surgeons found was that the clostridia infections could be classed in groups—important groups, for they determined both the type of treatment and the success that could be expected. First they found that many war wounds contained the microbes growing there as harmless guests, just as they might grow in a test tube in the laboratory. Whatever toxins they formed were discharged through the wounds immediately and lost, not absorbed into the body. Sometimes they grew so fast as to outgrow all other germs, but still they were just guests, nothing more.

What kept these germs from invading? Why did they attack one case and take a vacation on the tissues of another? Before answering that, let's take a look at the next class of patient they found. This was one whose wound was invaded slightly by the gas-forming germs. It was a little swollen, a little tender, perhaps a little painful, and sometimes there was a little hiss of escaping gas when the dressings were removed. Such findings meant almost certain amputation in World War I. Here was undeniable infection with the clostridia, but it certainly wasn't the fatal gas gangrene!

British surgeons laid these wounds wide open with the scalpel, probing into the deeper spaces where the germs seemed to lurk. They treated the patients at the same time with massive doses of the sulfa drugs and also with serum— remember, they didn't have penicillin then. They kept the wounds open and allowed in plenty of the oxygen that the bacteria didn't like. Almost all the patients got well without complication, showing that the infection couldn't have been very advanced, very deep inside the body. So now there was a second question. Why did some cases develop this simple sort of gas infection, which surgeons labeled "anaerobic cellulitis," an invasion of tissues by oxygen-hating germs?

The answer lay in some things the surgeons observed when they laid open those wounds that were only lightly invaded. One thing was always present, one observation characteristic. All contained dead tissues, usually muscle. Usually there wasn't much, but what there was showed definite evidence of attack by the germs. It was blackened, it was partially liquefied, its fibers were separated by bubbles of gas. Here, the British officers realized, was the beachhead by which the clostridia were able to attack the body.

The clinching point for this theory lay in the things surgeons observed in the real cases of gas gangrene, cases like those malignant ones seen in World War I, cases that, despite sulfonamides and potent serums, still died with about the same frequency they did twenty-odd years before on the battle-fields of France. They slashed open those wounds, too, and here they found great areas of devitalized muscle, foreign bodies that had not been removed, closed spaces that had not been properly opened. This was the picture, then, in real gas gangrene—widespread dead muscle, tissues that had lost their blood supply and were ripe victims for the Welch bacillus and its equally malignant brothers.

Now these British doctors had all the things necessary to formulate a real set of principles for preventing gas gangrene. But those principles had already been brought out. In the wounds of World War I it had been *débridement,* but the evacuation system had been slow then. Wounds that got back to the surgeon in a reasonable time got a thorough going-over, in some ways even more thorough than many of them get now, for the number of wounded was on a far greater scale in World War II than in anything that preceded it. But a lot of them didn't get back until the germs had already invaded the tissues, and neither the surgeon's scalpel nor the Dakin's irrigating tube, with its stream of chlorine-containing fluid, could reach them.

In the men from the Spanish Army, however, the ideal treatment had been generally carried out. They had been operated on soon after being wounded, in one of the small Hospitals of First Urgency placed just behind the front. The surgeons attacked the devitalized tissues before the germs that were always there had a chance to do their dirty work. And those surgeons had learned from a great master, for Trueta and his associates of the Republican Army Medical Service emphasized from the start that the answer to the whole problem lay in adequate surgery, not in plaster casts.

Adequate surgery and early surgery. It is like an oft-recurring strain of music, dinned into the ears of those surgeons just as it was dinned into the ears of our own American surgeons, until they knew nothing else, thought of nothing else. It meant cutting away all dead tissues, opening up wounds wide and leaving no deep pockets in which the germs of gas gangrene could begin gleefully to multiply and invade, keeping those wounds open but keeping out people and things that might further contaminate them.

Surgeons also dusted sulfa powder into the wounds in those days, but more and more thinking operators came to believe that it did but little good there and later its local use was discontinued. The powerful sulfa drugs were given by mouth, however, and when penicillin became available it was injected in large doses.

Surgery does not always reach the wounded man in time, however, and in the press of many casualties some devitalized tissue may be overlooked, some spaces that are not seen may be left behind as pockets in which the Welch bacillus and its equally evil brothers will grow. That is inevitable in the press of war time. That it happened only infrequently among American troops is ample evidence that mishaps occur only occasionally with an effective system of evacuation, front-line hospitals, and highly trained medical personnel. Certainly it was not the soil they were fighting over, for Africa, Sicily, Italy, France, and Germany were all highly cultivated areas.

What, then, can be offered the victim of gas gangrene? What hope is there for recovery? We would like to be able to give a sanguine answer, to say that gas gangrene as a disease has been done away with. And it is true that great inroads have been made against it, largely because of the powerful antibiotic drugs. But we still cannot say that a method of immunization has been perfected to protect soldiers against it as they are now protected against tetanus.

Immunization with tetanus toxoid in the months before battle, and activation of this immunity by an injection of the same preparation immediately after wounding, is truly one of the great sagas of the recent war. Who would have thought twenty years ago that in a conflict such as that, with millions of men locked in battle on every front, with thousands of great, dirt-infected wounds ripe for invasion by the slender, dark rods of the tetanus bacillus, the dread complications of lockjaw would not have to be feared any more? It is a disease of the past, a matter of military history.

While no such happy statement can be made about gas gangrene, it is true that penicillin and the other powerful antibiotics have given us an extremely formidable weapon against it. But the most important thing is what those Spanish wounded proved: the best way to treat the scourge is to remove its growing place. It's the same old story of success in saving wounded, the story told by pioneer Trueta back in the middle thirties: operate early and operate adequately.

But the story isn't finished. Surgeons at war are no different from their brothers in the laboratory, and they noted one encouraging thing about these early-treated wounds. Most of them didn't get infected at all. When the dressings were changed a week or ten days after the original operation, there was little or no inflammation. Early surgery and adequate surgery had removed the unhealthy tissue in which bacteria thrived. The obvious corollary was that now it was safe to close these wounds and promote rapid healing, to cut down the long period in which open wounds slowly filled in, to prevent the extensive scarring that follows such a filling in process.

Gradually, war surgeons began to close these healthy wounds secondarily, after all danger of infection was past. The results were amazingly successful, so successful that a new dictum of treatment could be set up. Clean wounds were closed with sutures, usually five to fifteen days after the original injury. Not only that but nerves could be repaired successfully then, and a certain amount of reconstructive surgery carried out very early in the history of the injury.

Hospitals were available for this work, fortunately, great general hospitals well back of the lines, staffed with highly trained specialists. They had equipment for carrying on unhurriedly the long, meticulous operations necessary to repair damaged nerves and blood vessels, ample facilities for blood transfusion, and plasma, everything that would be present in great university medical centers back in the States. In fact many of them were staffed by professors from these very university centers.

The results are now medical history. Undoubtedly this idea of leaving wounds open at first and closing them later will revolutionize civilian traumatic accident-surgery in the future. Again science and surgery have worked hand in hand on the battlefield and behind it, pointing the way to an even wider application in the years ahead.

But even while preparations were being made in the Laboratory for War that gave us the dictum of early and adequate surgery, science was attacking another of man's great scourges, peritonitis, laying the groundwork for results never before accomplished in treating wounds to which man is most vulnerable, those of the abdomen.

6.

PERITONITIS: THE CONQUEST OF A SCOURGE

What causes peritonitis—Old treatments—The Miller-Abbott tube—Blood proteins in peritonitis —Sulfa drugs and antibiotics—Other abdominal operations—Need of plasma

A great surgeon and teacher once told his students, "Know appendicitis and you know abdominal surgery." The abdomen is opened more frequently for the appendix than for perhaps all other conditions put together, and the abdomen is the most frequent site of surgery. Yet the ubiquitous little appendix may simulate any abdominal condition and cause more trouble than all the other abdominal organs together. For the surgeon to know abdominal surgery, he must first know appendicitis, and to know appendicitis, he must keep ever in mind the most frequently fatal complication of the inflamed appendix vermiformis, peritonitis.

In war and in peace, peritonitis is the enemy of the surgeon working inside the vitally important abdominal cavity. Wounds of the intestines always cause peritonitis, whether made by shrapnel, the surgeon's knife in resecting a cancer, or the rupture of the appendix or one of those tiny little appendixlike pockets called diverticulae. Fortunately, effective methods for the control of peritonitis have been devised. The way these methods were discovered and the way they work is one of the thrilling stories of modern surgical science.

As recently as the early thirties, appendicitis was taking a high death toll among its victims. Patients had not yet given up the accepted practice of taking a dose of castor oil for almost any sort of stomach ache, then calling the doctor some twenty-four hours later when the agony in their insides was beyond bearing and the delicate peritoneal membrane lining the abdominal cavity had become a tense, inflamed envelope, filled with the pus from a ruptured appendix.

Surgeons did one of two things then for those far-advanced cases. Either they operated at once and drained the inflamed abdomen, or they waited while the infection raged, building up the body resistance with transfusions, with fluid injected into the veins, and using slender rubber tubes to drain the stomach of the foul-smelling fluids that backed up from an intestinal tract powerless and immobilized by the dread "adynamic ileus" of peritonitis. Many cases died, but some localized the infection into abscesses; usually there was an abscess around the appendix but sometimes they were also found in the dozens of pockets and crevices of the lining membrane of the abdomen. These abscesses could be drained at operation, and the patients usually recovered, but only after a long, debilitating convalescence.

The results, generally speaking, were about the same whether the peritonitis cases were opened and drained at once or only after the abscesses had formed. The main difference seemed to be in the skill of those who directed the treatment, the tireless energy with which they fought on when there seemed no need to fight certain failure. In skilled hands only about five or ten peritonitis cases in every hundred died, but over the country the mortality was 20 to 25 per cent, often higher, as recently as fifteen years ago.

Meanwhile research scientists, laboratory specialists as well as surgeons, kept searching for facts to help control the often recurring disaster of peritonitis. They knew the cause of death in the cases that died. It lay in the strange paralysis of the intestinal tract that developed whether the patients were operated on immediately or treated by what were called "conservative methods." They called it "ileus," meaning intestinal obstruction, sometimes adding "adynamic" to signify that it was due to muscle paralysis.

Ileus didn't follow only appendicitis. It was common in intestinal wounds when the germ-teeming bowel contents escaped into the peritoneum and in perforations of the stomach from ulcer, as well as in almost any inflammation of the organs of the abdominal cavity. It even followed severe kidney-stone attacks, by a reflex process not entirely understood.

When the peritonitis cases were operated on the picture was the same, the abdomen tense, the peritoneum red and inflamed. Soon there was vomiting of a thick, dark, foul material, and the abdomen grew more and more distended while the patient became toxic and delirious, his skin dry from loss of fluids by vomiting. Too frequently this picture of intestinal paralysis went on to a fatal outcome.

No one could explain just what was happening to these peritonitis cases. Why should a patient who had no obstruction to the intestine behave exactly as if there were an obstruction? For this was the picture that older people called "lock bowels." Something did seem to be blocking the normal peristaltic waves of the muscle contraction in the intestinal wall, which push the contents on their way through the digestive tract.

For years surgeons had tried to combat ileus in many ways. They applied hot fomentations to the abdomen; they flogged the bowel with stimulating drugs such as pituitrin, which was supposed to make the muscles contract and set up peristalsis again. Irritating substances were injected into the large intestine in the hope of starting contractions in the small intestine that would sweep out the poisonous fluid and gas distending them. Sometimes these things helped; more often they didn't. Washing out the stomach with a tube seemed far better than anything else, but it was hard on a sick patient.

Then a better method of emptying the stomach was found in a small tube used in making gastric analysis. This tube could be passed through the nasal passages and kept in the stomach with suction applied. It stopped the constant vomiting and retching and seemed to relieve the absorption of poisons from the distended intestinal tract. Sometimes the tube passed through the stomach and into the small intestine, and then the patient often got rapidly better as the bowel was deflated.

This looked like a definite step in fighting ileus. Surgeons knew that when they could do this in an actual obstruction, the kind that came from adhesions, emptying the distended bowel made the patients get dramatically better, often allowed the obstruction to relieve itself and made further surgery unnecessary. They suspected that the same thing would happen with this paralytic obstruction that they called ileus.

Finally two searchers found the answer. Like every completely satisfactory solution to any perplexing problem, it turned out to be amazingly simple: a tube about ten feet long, with a partition down the middle—actually two tubes together. One side connected to a simple metal suction tip, just like any other stomach tube to which continuous suction is applied. The other connected to a small rubber balloon that could be inflated into a sausage-shaped structure around the end of the tube.

The Miller-Abbott tube is swallowed by the patient with the small balloon deflated, and is allowed to pass through the stomach into the first portion of the small intestine. The X-ray or fluoroscope shows when it is in place in the duodenum. Then the balloon is inflated with air, and the intestine seizes it, just as it would a portion of food, and pushes it down the alimentary canal. As it moves, the suction on the other side of the tube removes fluid and gas from the bowel ahead of it.

The tube thus keeps moving until it reaches the obstructed point. There it stops if the obstruction is complete, but more often relief of distension allows the intestine to disentangle itself and the obstruction is relieved. In ileus, deflation of the intestine allows it to take up its normal function once more.

One surgeon devised an ingenious method of getting the Miller-Abbott tube to pass into the small intestine, sometimes a rather difficult feat. Instead of putting air into the balloon at the outset, he put a small amount of mercury into it. The weight of the mercury pulled the end of the tube right down through the stomach and into the small intestine. Then by lowering the patient's head and raising the feet, thus putting the body on a slant, he caused the mercury to run out of the tube, after which air could be injected as usual.

The amazing change that occurs in the condition of a peritonitis victim when the distension poisoning his body is relieved, seems almost unbelievable. The Miller-Abbott tube is undeniably one of the greatest modern advances in the treatment of intestinal obstruction—whether mechanical or from intestinal paralysis.

But searchers didn't stop with this discovery. Another group were working on the problem of blood proteins. They knew that proteins disappeared rapidly from the blood in peritonitis, just as they did in shock, and they also knew that the material removed from distended intestines by the Miller-Abbott tube contained those very blood proteins that had been lost. On the basis of this, the answer soon became evident.

The pressure of gas in distended intestines causes a change in the tiny capillary blood vessels in the wall of the digestive tract. As a result, they are no longer able to hold the proteins in the blood stream. This lack of protein causes further fluid loss from the blood, and both together fill the distended intestine, setting up a vicious circle that becomes worse as the condition progresses. More fluid loss, more protein lack, more distension, and more protein loss—a never-ending chain. Relieving the distension with a rubber tube tackles this problem from the inside. Why not attack it also from the blood, they asked themselves, replacing lost fluids and proteins with plasma and blood transfusions?

This idea, too, proved to be sound. Keeping the blood proteins up with plasma and blood injection cut down the escape of fluid into the intestine. Thus there was less distension, less gas, and far less absorption of poisonous substances into the body. Sometimes building up blood protein relieves and prevents distension without a Miller-Abbott tube, but in severe cases both are used to good effect.

Now a method of combating the ileus of peritonitis had been found. If a way of combating the infection that caused it could be discovered, the peritonitis problem would be pretty well solved. That, too, was not long in the making.

Early in the development of the sulfa drugs it was evident that these chemicals were very effective against the germs that usually cause peritonitis. In laboratories it had been shown already that the germs that cause the disease could be whittled down to two main groups, the "colon group" and the "streptococcus group," with sometimes another particularly malignant invader, the "gas-gangrene group," headed by the fat, dark-staining Welch bacillus.

Sulfanilamide was already known to be effective against these germs. Why not use it in appendicitis?

So the peritonitis fighters set up experiments in which they created appendicitis in laboratory animals. The control group were left without any protection; practically all of them died. Others got injections of the new drugs, both before the operation and after. And here a wonderful thing happened. Those animals who got the drug lived a lot longer—and most miraculous of all, many of them recovered. The evidence was plain; sulfanilamide protected to a certain extent at least against the germs of peritonitis resulting from a ruptured appendix.

This was but a wedge in the drive to split the peritonitis front wide open, but it was driven home quickly by other searchers. Since sulfanilamide protected the animals against experimental appendicitis, why wouldn't it protect humans? No experimental animals were needed here, no volunteers such as made possible the epoch-making discoveries of Walter Reed with yellow fever. Every day a stream of unfortunate victims of that treacherous little organ poured through hospitals.

They came into the great University of Pennsylvania Hospital, and there they got the best treatment available at that time. They got that and something else, for a group of surgeons here was at work on the peritonitis problem.

Patients with peritonitis couldn't take sulfanilamide by mouth, so an ingenious way of getting the drug into the body was devised. It was dissolved in a dilute solution, then allowed to run slowly into the tissues beneath the skin until a substantial dose had been injected. It had to be given that way because the drug could not be injected into the veins in that form.

Results were at once apparent. Patients had less trouble, they recovered more quickly, and mortality rates were definitely lowered. Remember, this was before the days of powerful antibiotics such as penicillin and the "-mycin" group.

And then one day a young surgeon in Memphis opened up a case of peritonitis. It was a messy affair, the intestines bathed in pus, their surfaces already furry with the exudate that so often ties up the bowel even after the sick person has recovered from the infection itself, causing frequent attacks of dangerous intestinal obstruction. Surgeons had been pouring sulfanilamide into dirty automobile-accident wounds for many months; most of the reports indicated that it was highly effective in controlling infection in these cases, whether from any local effect or from a general effect, no one yet knew. If any wound deserved direct application of the drug this one did, but nobody before then had tried dumping it into the peritoneum, or at least they hadn't reported it in the medical literature.

So he took a chance and poured sulfanilamide into this peritoneal cavity, closed up the wound, and watched anxiously for some sign of beneficial effect. The signs were quick to develop. The patient soon turned blue, but that was to be expected, for most patients who took sulfanilamide turned blue. The next three or four days would tell the tale. Ordinarily the sick man's temperature would rise, his abdomen would become distended and hard with the adynamic ileus of peritonitis.

And what happened this time? Besides the expected blueness—nothing. Temperature dropped to normal almost immediately. There was no distension, no tense, rigid abdomen, no toxicity. In fact, this patient didn't seem any different from a dozen others scattered through the ward whose appendices had not ruptured.

It seemed easy to figure what had happened. The sulfanilamide was obviously absorbed from the peritoneum into the blood stream, as witness the blue color, just as it would be absorbed from tissues anywhere if a solution was injected into them. Suppose, then, that in the process of absorption very high concentrations of sulfanilamide occurred in the tissues of the abdomen, concentrations so high that they not only attacked the ordinary germs that the drug destroyed but also a lot of others that it did not ordinarily affect. That, too, seemed reasonable to a lot of people.

As always proves the case, it now appears that much of the enthusiasm for the use of sulfonamide drugs in the peritoneum, and also in wounds, was not quite justified. Newer sulfonamides—much more effective against many more germs and with much lower blood concentrations of the drug—plus the powerful antibiotic groups, have done away with the necessity of pouring it into the peritoneum and into dirty wounds to get it into the body very quickly.

The groundwork had been done, largely with the problem of appendicitis. Now a greater testing laboratory was being developed, for the world was in the beginnings of a great war. And war meant abdominal wounds, the worst disaster that can happen to the soldier on the battlefield.

Wounds involving the abdomen have always been the most dangerous of all war-time injuries. World War I showed a mortality rate of about 60 per cent in severe abdominal wounds. The reason for this high death rate is not hard to see. The abdomen contains many of the body's most vital organs. There are the great blood vessels, the aorta and the vena cava, and the many important branches of both, severance of which by bullet or shell fragment means not only the strong possibility of death from hemorrhage alone, but the destruction from lack of blood of the organs these vessels supply.

There are solid organs in the abdomen, too—the liver, spleen, kidneys, pancreas. Many of these produce a secretion intensely irritating if it escapes into the peritoneal cavity. And most dangerous of all, of course, there is the gastrointestinal tract, the organs of the alimentary canal, teeming with bacteria, the same bacteria that cause the familiar picture of peritonitis in civilian life from perforation of the inflamed appendix or penetrating stomach ulcer.

Considering all these sources of trouble, it is not hard to understand that the two most pressing dangers in an abdominal wound are shock with hemorrhage—always inseparable—and peritonitis. The answer to lowering mortality from these wounds, then, seems to lie in controlling these two factors.

Surgeons of the Spanish War, the pioneers in the vast laboratory of conflict, realized that if they were to treat abdominal wounds successfully they must tackle these two problems. But tackling them successfully meant operating early, before hemorrhage exhausted the wounded soldier and before the poisonous bowel contents had too freely invaded the sensitive peritoneal lining of the abdomen.

Spanish surgeons formulated a simple rule for treatment.

It wasn't the skill of the surgeon that counted so much, provided he knew enough to open an abdomen, search it thoroughly, stop hemorrhage, and close bowel perforations. The most important thing was that these wounds be operated on within the six hours after wounding. And before the operation, while operating, and afterward, blood transfusions or injections of blood plasma must be kept running into the injured man's veins. They were combating at the operating table the two great hazards, shock-with-hemorrhage and contamination from bowel perforations by bullet or shell.

Now we can begin to understand how perspiring medical officers in the jungles of New Guinea achieved miracles in saving abdominal-wound cases. They were working in a small area, practically in the front lines, for sometimes those hospitals had to spend almost as much time dodging Japanese snipers as they did operating. They got their patients in time to control the hemorrhage and treat the shock with blood and plasma, and in time to operate and close the perforations before there was much chance of peritoneal soiling. And then they followed up with the many methods of trouble prevention developed in the last twenty years, particularly the all-important sulfa drugs, the Miller-Abbott tube, blood plasma, transfusions, and penicillin.

From war-time experience came a definite regime for handling abdominal wounds. The first thing was to get the patient early. That meant putting hospitals close to the front, or if this was impossible, widespread use of air evacuation to rush the wounded back to a hospital at the earliest possible moment. The value of this was shown particularly during the more recent Korean conflict.

Along with these went measures to control the first important factor, hemorrhage. Plasma was given all the way down the line from the very foxholes to the hospital, and once at the hospital, blood, too, was given. Generally, in severe hemorrhage, surgeons estimated that lost blood could be replaced in the ratio of about equal parts of plasma and blood. But if more was available for transfusions, it was given.

The British forces at Tobruk showed the way. Before every major attack they built up a blood bank from their convalescent patients, hospital corpsmen, volunteer donors all. Then when the wounded started pouring in they were ready.

An abdominal case arriving at the hospital was quickly evaluated. If he needed plasma or blood before operation, it was given, usually while the operation was going on, for frequently it was impossible to bring a wounded man completely out of shock before operation. His condition improved quickly after the source of the hemorrhage had been located and controlled.

Operation was performed and the abdomen thoroughly explored. Bleeding areas were controlled and perforations in the stomach and intestines closed. Openings in the large intestine, it was found, should be exteriorized, brought out through the incision, in a manner familiar to all surgeons from the "Mikulicz" operation for cancer.

At that time most surgeons dusted sulfa powder into the peritoneum before closing the abdominal wall with a few sutures. Now we know, with the tremendously more effective antibiotics that we have today, even these wounds can be closed and infection prevented at the very beginning.

Nor did military surgeons wait for peritonitis, for distension, for vomiting, to occur in their abdominal-wound cases. Given an early operation, and plenty of sulfonamide treatment, they knew, many cases would not develop peritonitis at all, but they still didn't take chances. They continued to inject sulfadiazine into the veins and penicillin into the muscles to keep up a strong concentration of the vital germ-killing drugs in the blood stream. They put down the Miller-Abbott tube because they knew it would pass through the stomach much more easily before actual vomiting started. And they knew, too, that if they kept the intestine from becoming dilated there would be less loss of protein and less probability of an adynamic ileus, with a better chance for the patient to come through. The tube was placed well into the small intestine and a constant suction kept on it so as to abort any distension that might begin. In addition, fluid intake was maintained by injecting sugar and salt solution into the veins and, most important of all, blood plasma and transfusions to build up the protein.

By doing these things early, military surgeons averted most

of the distressing effects of abdominal injuries and they avoided the period of agony and waiting while a patient fights his battle against peritonitis unaided.

This regime of expectant treatment is yielding results in civilian surgical practice. Surgeons no longer wait with their appendix patients who have gone on to perforation. They treat these cases in which infection has blown a hole in the wall of the appendix just as military surgeons treat damage to the bowel from outside sources, by protecting from ileus and by warding off the dangers of obstruction.

Obstructions from adhesions and other sources will still develop, but no longer do surgeons have to rush poorly prepared patients to the table for emergency operations. With the Miller-Abbott tube, blood proteins, plus sulfa, penicillin, and the other antibiotic drugs, it is usually safe to relieve the obstruction from the inside first and to build up the patient's condition before operating. Often operation is not necessary after those things have been done.

Here again science and surgery are working together, to fight peritonitis and obstruction, the two greatest dangers in abdominal operations. In so doing they have made safer operations on other abdominal organs, particularly in those great new fields in which science has contributed so much to make surgery possible, the liver and the pancreas.

7.

PROTEINS AND PROTHROMBIN

*The liver and its functions—The gall bladder—
Gallstones and surgery—Vitamin K and clotting
of blood—Production of prothrombin—Surgery of
the liver and gall bladder •*

To the consistent radio and TV fan, the liver is familiar as an organ with a habit of sleeping, continually needing "waking up" by the advertised brand of tiny brown pellets; periodically, under the stimulus of drugs, it empties itself of "liver bile," thus turning a sour, complaining individual into a picture of optimism and *joie de vivre*. Fortunately, medical science has carried the study of the liver and its ailments a great deal further than this, and as usual it has called on the other sciences to aid in the search for truth. Surgeons use this knowledge in their own work on the liver. The lowered mortality rate from liver, bile-duct, and gall-bladder surgery, and the increasingly satisfactory results obtained, all bear witness to the thoroughness of the search.

The liver is in every sense an indispensable organ. Damage to it is immediately reflected in the function of every other part of the body. This essentialness of an organ, about which the average person knows practically nothing (an ignorance shared largely by medical science until the past few decades), derives from a number of vital functions it performs, functions that govern the action and life of almost every cell of the body. To understand how modern surgery approaches diseases of the liver and its component parts, one must understand first the position it occupies in the body, and second, the manifold functions it performs.

69

Anatomically, the liver is a filtration plant between the gastrointestinal tract, from which the digested food is absorbed, and the general blood stream. All veins from the upper portion of the digestive tract join together to form a large vessel, the portal vein, which passes into the liver. Here the food material finds itself inside a busy factory manufacturing many products. Let us look for a second into a single unit of this factory.

The unit of function as well as structure in the liver is a tiny portion of tissue called a lobule. Thinking for the moment of the lobule as a square of liver cells, we find a branch of the portal vein at each corner of the square, pouring food-laden blood from the digestive tract into the lobule. The food-laden blood passes toward the center of the square, bathing the liver cells as it goes. At the center of the lobule another vein picks up the blood and carries it on its way throughout the body. Between the corners of the lobule and its center many things have happened, and on these changes the function of the liver depends.

First is the effect on carbohydrates. Carbohydrates are broken up by the digestive tract into simple sugars, called dextrose or glucose. Glucose is pure sugar and circulates as such. But if all the sugar taken into the body were to stay in the blood there would be a flooding of all cells with sugar three times a day, and between times the level would fall to a point at which the functions of the vital and delicate brain cells might be seriously endangered. To keep the level of sugar in the blood always at a safe point, the body stores this sugar in the liver. This is done by a complex physico-chemical change whereby the simple glucose becomes a more concentrated substance called glycogen. This glucose-to-glycogen change in the liver is governed by another substance produced in the pancreas called insulin.

Insulin acts as a governor of glucose in the body. Cut down the production of insulin and sugar accumulates in the blood. Not only that, but the use of fat in the body is seriously interfered with in the absence of the proper metabolism of sugar.

It is a physiological maxim taught to medical students that "fats burn in the fire of the carbohydrates, without them they smoke." So without proper use of carbohydrate-sugars because of poor insulin production, the fats form dangerous by-products of an acid nature, and in severe cases acidosis with coma and death may ensue. Most people are familiar with this story, for it is that of diabetes, the disease that formerly caused many deaths but is now controlled by the injection of insulin.

The glucose-controlling functions of the liver are only a part of its manifold job, however. It also acts as a policeman to the blood, singling out poisonous or toxic substances that may have been absorbed along with the food and attempting to destroy them before they enter the general circulation and reach the delicate and very sensitive cells of the brain and other organs. Sometimes these substances are too strong for the liver and it is damaged by them. Years ago this was a rather common occurrence with chloroform, a drug now known to be so dangerous because of its effects on the liver that its use as an anesthetic has been largely given up by most surgeons.

The liver, too, functions in the use of proteins by the body. Protein foods, such as meats and milk, are digested in the stomach and small intestine into simple units called amino acids. These amino acids can be used by the body for energy, just as glucose is used, but first the nitrogen they contain must be split off and removed lest the by-products formed by burning amino acids for energy also act as poisons to the body.

The process of de-aminization, or splitting away of nitrogen from protein foods, is carried out in the liver. From this chemical reaction, a substance called urea is formed, which is subsequently thrown off by the kidneys. If the liver function for protein de-poisoning falls down, however, poisonous by-products, such as urea, begin to accumulate in the blood and serious effects occur.

But de-aminization is not the sole work of the liver cells with protein foods, for the liver factory turns out still another product, individual body protein. We eat meat in the form of steak, but for it to become part of our own muscle, it must first be digested as amino acids, and then these acids must be put together like a jigsaw puzzle to form our own body protein, in a series of complicated chemical reactions that have not yet been duplicated in the laboratory, though the ubiquitous liver does it easily.

These are functions enough for any organ, but the liver lobule has just begun to work. Not only does it utilize the digested food, it helps digest it, too. This digestive function depends on another product of liver activity, a brown fluid called bile. Bile acts on the fats to aid in their digestion. Liver cells in the process of their work manufacture bile.

Between the strands of liver cells extending from the corner of the liver lobule to the center, there are tiny tubes called bile capillaries. These tubes collect the bile formed by individual liver cells and, running from lobule to lobule, gather it together into ever larger tubes, like the branches of a tree. Finally two great trunks, one from each side of the liver, join into a single tube, called the "common bile duct." This duct empties into the first portion of the small intestine, the duodenum, roughly three to five inches beyond the stomach.

Through the bile capillaries and the bile ducts, a continuous stream of bile trickles to aid in digestion. But here again we are faced with the fact that the digestive tract is stoked with food three times a day. For large quantities of bile to be available when the intestine fills with food for thrice-daily digestion, there should be a reservoir to hold the bile between times. It is there, a pear-shaped pouch lying beneath the liver and connected to the side of the common bile duct by a smaller tube called the cystic duct. This reservoir is the gall bladder, and it is here that the surgeon's troubles really begin.

Bile accumulates in the gall bladder and regularly, stimulated by the presence of food—particularly fats, which cannot be digested without bile—empties itself into the common bile duct and thus into the duodenum, the first portion of the intestine. But because the bile lies stagnant in the gall bladder for varying periods of time, strange things sometimes happen.

Nobody knows for sure which comes first, infection or gall stones. Most surgeons think the gall bladder must be infected by germs from some other source before the bile begins to solidify into stones. Others think the gall stones precede the infection. Whichever way it happens, small stones occur and sometimes the gall bladder fills up with them.

Now comes trouble. If the stones are large or if there is

only a single large stone, there may be nothing but occasional mild stomach aches and a form of indigestion causing fullness and discomfort after eating greasy foods, which is characteristic of gall-bladder disease. But if the stones are small enough to slip into the narrow cystic duct leading from the gall bladder to the common bile duct, things happen rapidly. The stones lodge in the duct, and the gall bladder tries to force them down by contracting. The result is a severe, sharp pain, which usually darts through the body and may locate under the right shoulder blade. The pain is terrific and is known as "gall-bladder colic."

Once the colic starts two things may happen. The stone may be forced through the narrow cystic duct and enter the much larger common bile duct. Often the stone escapes into the intestine, where it becomes harmless. But let the stone block the common bile duct and trouble really begins. This obstruction to the main bile passage is the most difficult problem of liver and bile-duct surgery. Most frequently it is seen after gall-bladder operations in which a stone has been overlooked.

But why operate on the gall bladder at all, if the stones inside it do not actually obstruct the passage of bile down the common bile duct? The reasoning here is similar to that followed in appendicitis.

Block off the appendix by material escaping from the bowel into its narrow inside passage and it begins to swell, becomes inflamed, and eventually may rupture. Block the duct from the gall bladder with a stone and the same thing happens. The gall bladder becomes tense with bile, swelling increases. Somewhere along the line the swelling shuts off the flow of blood to the arteries of the gall-bladder wall, and gangrene of the pouch occurs. The wall of the gall bladder then breaks, the infection spills out, and peritonitis or an abscess results. Meanwhile the patient has become desperately ill and unless the diagnosis is made and operation performed to remove or drain the gall bladder, death may ensue. Surgeons are coming more and more to believe that an acutely obstructed and inflamed gall bladder is as much of an emergency as an acute appendix or a perforated ulcer of the stomach. This approach is already paying dividends in lives saved.

So much for the gall bladder. What of the stone that blocks the flow of bile through the common bile duct? This is the problem that keeps surgeons awake nights, for once the flow of bile becomes obstructed, a dangerous sequence of events sets in, leading to practically certain death unless the obstruction is relieved in some way.

Blocking the common bile duct is like damming a flowing stream. The pressure back of the dam accumulates and is reflected along ever smaller branches of the stream. Eventually it backs up into the bile capillaries in the liver lobules themselves, and then is absorbed into the blood.

Once bile appears in appreciable quantities in the blood, jaundice occurs, the eyeballs become yellow, the skin takes on a saffron hue and begins to itch intolerably, and the patient becomes acutely miserable and ill. As if this weren't enough, he may find himself bleeding seriously from minor cuts and scratches. If a tyro surgeon is so ill-advised as to operate without the proper preliminary tests, the jaundiced patient may bleed to death on the operating table.

This bleeding tendency depends on still another property of the liver, that having to do with the clotting of the blood. A few years ago scientists discovered a new substance they called vitamin K. They found that this vitamin, when absorbed in the diet and taken into the body, caused the liver to form another fascinating substance, with the name of prothrombin.

There was a catch to this, though, for unless there was bile in the intestine, sent there by a properly functioning liver, the vitamin K was not absorbed and prothrombin was not manufactured. It was a little like a dog chasing its tail. Bile formed by the liver enabled the body to take in vitamin K, which then formed prothrombin in the liver along with more bile.

This process of manufacturing prothrombin was until recently one of the least-understood functions of the liver, yet it is now known to be probably the most important of all. For without prothrombin, another substance, thrombin, cannot be formed. And without thrombin acting on the liquid portion of the blood, no clots will occur. So if you have no prothrombin and you cut yourself, you may bleed to death.

This fact explains the bleeding tendency in jaundice. Bile cannot reach the intestine, therefore vitamin K cannot be absorbed, *ergo*, the liver does not form prothrombin, and bleeding occurs.

The answer would seem simple. Operate and relieve the obstruction to the bile, then the process will reverse itself and everything will be all right.

But there was a hitch to that, too. How could you operate to relieve the tendency to hemorrhage, if you couldn't control bleeding from your operative incision? For a long time surgeons got around this problem to a certain extent by injecting calcium, which helped to make the blod clot, and more important, by giving blood transfusions, which gave an injection of prothrombin into the sick person's blood stream. By operating now and, if there was any bleeding tendency, continuing to give blood, the surgeon could tide the patient over until he could absorb his own vitamin K and form his own supply of vital prothrombin. It was an ingenious application of what scientists had learned about the liver and the blood; and it worked—most of the time.

But however ingenious the idea, it wasn't perfect and something else was needed. That substance turned up in the form of a chemical with a jawbreaker of a name, 2-methyl-1, 4 naphthoquinone. This was simply synthetic vitamin K, a chemical that could be injected into the body, whereupon the liver took it and formed its own prothrombin. The discovery of this chemical was a great step forward in liver surgery and meant that surgeons could operate on a lot of miserable common-duct obstruction cases they formerly hadn't been able to do very much about.

But one thing troubled surgeons still. Some of their severe jaundice patients went on and died anyway, although the operation was correctly performed, the obstruction relieved, and the patients given those two extremely important benefits, adequate pre- and post-operative treatment.

So doctors began to search for some way to estimate the ability of a given patient's liver to stand the shock of an operation and just how much recuperative power it possessed to build itself back up to normal after the long drain of not functioning properly.

Fortunately, pharmacologists had many years before worked out a method of looking into livers and gall bladders with the X-ray; they gave the patient a drug that appears in the bile and fills up the gall bladder, making it visible on an X-ray film. In a way this is also a test of liver and gall-bladder function. Surgical researchers in liver disease now wondered why it wouldn't be possible to inject one of these liver-selective drugs into the blood and then measure the rate at which it disappeared as it was excreted from the liver as bile. They used tetra-bromphenolphthaleïn, a first cousin of the X-ray chemical, and found that it did give a fairly good idea of how the liver was working, though it wasn't a perfect test.

Now, your true scientist doesn't give up because his first attempt, or his first hundred or thousand attempts, don't produce the result he is looking for. He keeps on searching, and his very persistence has given us such discoveries as insulin, penicillin, and a host of other boons to mankind. All over the world medical scientists were searching for a good liver-function test. Many were used, some of them good.

Then Dr. A. J. Quick and his co-workers managed to find a satisfactory method of measuring the prothrombin in the blood. Here was something for a start. Prothrombin was low when the liver was not functioning well, either from lack of vitamin K or from damage by long-standing obstruction or infection. That was known to be true. Inject vitamin K, synthetically formed in the chemist's laboratory by this time, into a person with a working liver, and prothrombin was shortly built up to a normal level. *Ergo,* test liver function by measuring the rate at which it formed prothrombin from injected vitamin K. Now they were getting somewhere, and time has proved the value of their work.

Given a jaundice case from an obstruction of the bile ducts by stones, the surgeon goes methodically about finding out just what shape his patient is in. First he measures the jaundice index, which tells him just how bad the bile back-up is. Then he measures the prothrombin index, which tells him how badly the liver is failing to perform its normal functions. Along with this he studies the blood proteins, so important in shock, and the chlorides and the cholesterol concentrations, which we know now also reflect the general condition of the patient's liver function. But above all, he injects synthetic vitamin K, or gives large doses of it by mouth along with bile salts so that it will be properly absorbed. Then on succeeding days he tests the blood prothrombin to find out just what the liver is doing.

If the prothrombin comes promptly back up to normal, the surgeon knows that the function of the patient's liver has been only temporarily interfered with by the obstruction to the passage of bile, and that when the obstruction is relieved at operation, recovery will promptly ensue. But if there is a delay in forming prothrombin or if it fails to rise, the surgeon takes a graver view. Such findings indicate a damaged liver, and he must proceed much more cautiously.

These unfortunate individuals he will not immediately bring to the operating table. Instead he will put them on a diet high in carbohydrates and proteins, with plenty of calories and plenty of vitamins. He will inject glucose and give transfusions of fresh, strong blood from healthy donors. When these measures have been taken, the surgeon again checks the function of the liver, and when it seems best, he operates. But he's even more careful after operation to keep the strength of these liver patients right up to normal, to keep always ahead of trouble, for keeping ahead means saving lives—the surgeon's job.

All this emphasis on what might be called pure science with regard to liver disease might make one think that operative technique and the skill of the surgeon, born of years of study and training, are the least important items in successful liver surgery. Nothing could be further from the truth. When working on a vital organ like the liver, there can be no compromises. Damage its function seriously for much more than a matter of hours and all the surgical skill in the world is of no avail, so only highly trained surgeons attempt the delicate operations on the bile ducts that are often the only way of saving lives.

Gall-bladder surgery centers usually in the question of stones. Inflammation of the gall bladder in the absence of stones does occur, but only rarely. More often the sequence of events is that already described; a stone attempts to work its way down the cystic (gall-bladder) duct and gets stuck there. Pain follows immediately, with inflammation and possibly gangrene and perforation.

Surgeons tackle these acute cases in two ways. Some prefer to operate immediately, or after a short period of preparation, just as a surgeon often takes time to build up even an acute appendix case by injecting glucose into the veins and perhaps building up a buffer of the proper antibiotic in the blood. More and more surgeons are coming to believe that patients do better when diseased and acutely obstructed gall bladders are removed as soon as the diagnosis can be made.

This emphasis on early operation is in sharp contrast to the second method, practiced by most surgeons up to about two decades ago. Gall-bladder disease was treated then by waiting and operating only after repeated attacks. This tendency to wait stemmed partially from a very natural reluctance to take out the bile reservoir for fear of secondary effects from its lack. There is no denying that such effects do follow the removal of the normal gall bladder, but the surgeon is dealing here with the lesser of two evils. No gall bladder at all is better than one that is causing pain and recurrently becoming inflamed. A fact not considered often enough, even by enlightened surgeons, is that each attack of gall-bladder colic and inflammation undoubtedly damages the liver a little bit, still another reason why there was little point in leaving in an already damaged gall bladder.

But not every case of indigestion from eating fatty foods is gall-bladder disease, it should be pointed out. To remove a normal gall bladder from a case of nervous indigestion of the type that is becoming more and more frequent with the tension of modern life, is only going to make bad matters worse, very much worse. For this reason surgeons wholeheartedly condemn the practice, not infrequent still, of removing gall bladders because they are to a certain extent a superfluous organ. It is true that the common bile duct does become dilated after gall-bladder removal and does to a certain degree take over the reservoir function of the gall bladder, but a normal gall bladder is still decidedly better than none at all.

When the common bile duct becomes blocked, from stones,

from inflammation in its vicinity, or from operations on the gall bladder, problems arise that truly try the souls of conscientious surgeons. We have seen how the liver is affected by obstructions of this type and how its function can be evaluated by special tests. We have seen, too, how the surgeon goes about preparing his patients for operation with injections of vitamin K, blood transfusions, plasma injections, or the new simplified protein foods, amino acids, which can be injected along with the glucose so necessary to protect the liver from the exigencies of the anesthetic and the operation. When the surgeon takes his scalpel in hand, it is his own skill that guards the patient against trouble and that insures a happy result, his own skill again bulwarked by science and the products of the laboratory.

The most common obstruction to the common bile duct is from stones, either formed at the time similar obstructing pebbles are formed in the gall bladder, overlooked at the time of gall-bladder surgery, or occurring secondarily after gall-bladder removal. Operation here, though meticulous and trying because of the scar tissue so often present where there have been previous operations, is not too difficult.

First the surgeon locates the common bile duct; usually it is dilated and therefore easier to find. Then he opens it, cleans out the stones, and inserts an ingenious rubber tube in the shape of a T, which allows bile to pass through the intestine but still has an escape passage to the outside. He lets the excess bile drain, often for weeks after the operation, until the liver function is well established again. If there is any doubt that the bile ducts are wide open, he injects a chemical through the tube and takes an X-ray, thus visualizing the inside of the liver and its duct system. When everything is clear, the tube is removed and the wound allowed to heal.

Where there has been damage to the common bile duct, the operation becomes many times more serious. It may be necessary then to remove the strictured area and sew the duct together again without the constriction. Ingenious tubes of an inert metal, vitallium, have been devised that can be inserted as a mold around which a new duct forms. If nothing else, a rubber tube can be inserted directly into the liver ducts and bile drained out through the operative wound.

Gradually there forms a tube from the liver to the skin, called an "external biliary fistula," from which bile pours. Later a small rubber catheter is inserted into this tube-fistula tract and it is carefully dissected away from the abdominal wall until there is a tube some three to six inches long connected to the liver, and taking the place of the original damaged bile duct.

Turning this fistula around and attaching the former skin opening to the intestine smacks of a surgical miracle, but it is performed regularly by skilled surgeons. The new artificial bile duct works perfectly in many cases, and the bile reaches its original objective once more. There are many ways to replace damaged bile ducts, all of them results of ingenious applications of scientific principles to liver surgery.

As with many other of the vital organs of the body, such as the heart, the frontiers of liver surgery are constantly being pushed back, and there is no doubt that more extensive operations on the liver will be performed as time goes on. Meanwhile a neighboring organ, the pancreas, is also yielding to the surgeon's scalpel, bulwarked with the discoveries of modern medical science.

8.

SWEETBREADS AND SUGAR TOLERANCE

> *The pancreas, its double life—The islands of Langerhans—Diabetes—Insulin—Operating on diabetics—Excess insulin—Tumor of the pancreas—Cancer of the pancreas meant sure death twenty years ago—The delicate operation used now—Grafting pancreatic tissue into diabetics—Transplanting of complete organs*

Deep inside the body nestles a small, pennant-shaped organ that because of its very inaccessibility has long baffled surgeons—the pancreas, in animals called sweetbreads.

Until the last decade, surgery of the pancreas was practically unknown, attempted only by a few exceptionally skilled operators. So rapid, however, has been progress in our knowledge of this little-known organ that within the past five years whole volumes have been written on the surgical treatment of diseases of the pancreas.

Thousands of lives will be saved in years to come because of the persistence and daring of a few pioneer surgeons.

The pancreas occupies the somewhat unique position of being a gland of both external and internal secretions. This means simply that it is really two organs in one. Scientists studying this organ learned the strange double life of the pancreas a long time ago, when they looked at microscopic sections of its anatomical structure.

Outwardly it is a gland like the liver, or the salivary glands, which swell up and become painful when you get the mumps. Like them it has a system of tubes arranged like the branches of a tree to carry the substances manufactured in the gland

and empty them into the digestive tract. Glands such as this are called glands of external secretion, because they manufacture substances that are then poured out through the tubular ducts. The secretion formed by the pancreas is largely trypsin, an active agent in the digestion of proteins.

Recently trypsin has begun to be more widely used in medicine because of its ability to digest dead tissues. At present, treatment with this particular drug is in a somewhat experimental state, but the omens seem to be that it will be a valuable addition to medical science in the future.

Glands of internal secretion, commonly called endocrine or ductless glands, are quite different. They have no tube system and no secretion is carried off and emptied outside the gland. Instead, the cells of the ductless glands are bathed continuously in blood from the network of tiny blood vessels surrounding them. The substances formed by these cells, called hormones, are taken directly into the blood stream and carried all over the body, exerting profound effects on the working of practically every individual body cell.

Take for example the thyroid, perhaps the most familiar of the ductless glands. If something goes wrong with it, a swelling occurs in the neck, called a goiter, which sometimes has to be removed at operation. If the thyroid gets lazy, you become sluggish, sleepy, mentally slowed down, your face swells, and your metabolism rate goes down. If it works too fast, you are overalert and nervous, lose weight, your metabolism goes up, as does your pulse—the picture known as hyperthyroidism.

Now, the pancreas didn't look like a gland of internal secretion to early anatomists. It had a duct, and it poured its digestive juice into the intestine. But when the anatomists cut thin slices of tissue, stained them, and looked at the cells under the microscope, they found a strange thing. Part of the gland was just as they had expected, the familiar picture of glands such as this, with nests of cells hollow inside, resembling grapes with hollow stems, the ducts. All glands of external secretion have much the same structure.

But between these nests of normal gland cells there were other groups, foreign cells that seemed to have no particular purpose. They were arranged in islands and had no ducts.

If they manufactured anything, it must be absorbed directly into the blood stream. The anatomist who first discovered these strange groups of cells was honored by having his name attached to them, and they are called the islands of Langerhans. It was obvious that the island cells had some function, but no one knew exactly what it was.

Then toward the end of the last century investigators searching for the facts about this little-known organ, tried to remove it completely from animals. The animals recovered, foretelling our modern operations on the pancreas in humans, but a peculiar thing happened, a thing that was completely unexplainable at the time. The animals all got diabetes.

Now, diabetes was not a new disease. The Greeks had known about it a few thousand years before and people had gone on dying from it over the years. Ancient physicians knew that sugar wasn't properly used by the body in diabetes. They knew, too, that much of the sugar was excreted in the urine, giving it a sweet taste and attracting bees and flies. But of all the theories postulated to explain diabetes, the nearest explanation up to that time was that the disturbance of sugar utilization occurred in the liver. They weren't too far wrong even at that, for the substance that prevents diabetes, insulin, is known to act largely on the liver.

From the evidence at hand investigators concluded that the pancreas produced a substance that controlled the use of sugar in the body, a substance whose absence produced diabetes. Even then some doubters thought the damage to nerves in removing the pancreas might have caused the effect. It remained only to prove that if one removed the pancreas and then transplanted a portion of it in another part of the body, diabetes didn't occur.

The next logical step was to extract a substance from the pancreas, removed from experimental animals, that could then be used to prevent diabetes in those same animals. These attempts failed, but so confident were the searchers that they were on the right track that the undiscovered substance was even named. It was called "insuline," because it was recognized that it was produced in the islands of Langerhans.

The reason searchers for the potent extract of pancreas tissue failed is easy to understand now. Insulin is a protein, and since the trypsin produced by the pancreas is an active digester of protein, the extract was being digested as fast as it was made. Things remained in pretty much this state of impasse until 1922, when Banting and Best succeeded in a tricky experiment. They operated on animals and tied off the duct from the pancreas. The trypsin-forming cells then dried up—the medical word is atrophied—leaving the island cells behind. From these island cells they extracted insulin, with historic results.

Surgery can do little for diabetics, although modern knowledge of that disease has done miracles in assisting the surgeon when it becomes necessary to operate on the diabetic patient. Here the diabetic specialist and the surgeon work hand in hand, and many a limb has been saved because of that close co-operation. Infections always make diabetes worse, too, and by means of the same close partnership between medical specialist and surgeon, great steps have been made in combating this ever dangerous complication in the diabetic.

To the surgeon the most fascinating problem related to the pancreas is a strange and dramatic sort of thing that is the very reverse of diabetes. Insulin lowers the sugar of the body, preventing the effects of diabetes. But keep on injecting insulin and the blood sugar goes on down. Soon the patient becomes unconscious; a little later convulsions set in. Continue the injection and death will ensue.

Psychiatrists use this excess insulin reaction to treat mental disease, lowering the blood sugar until they receive the effect they wish, then pumping sugar into the stomach to overcome the action of the insulin or, in an emergency, giving it into the veins. They often achieve remarkable effects on mental disease, sometimes using smaller amounts of insulin that do not actually cause a convulsion.

Occasionally doctors saw patients who exhibited the same sort of phenomenon without taking insulin. Many of them had already learned that they could avoid these fainting and convulsion attacks by eating sugar. They even carried the sugar with them everywhere they went, to be ready. The laboratory showed that these patients needed sugar, too, for if the blood was tested when one of the attacks was coming on, it showed a very low sugar level. Some of these people died, either from the attacks or from a peculiar type of malignant tumor. When their bodies were studied at the post mortem examination, tumors of the pancreas were found.

The pancreas is subject to the formation of several kinds of tumors. Any gland forms fluid-filled sacs called cysts, and surgeons have long recognized such tumors in the pancreas. They recognized, too, that these cysts of the pancreas contained a large amount of trypsin. If they were opened and the fluid escaped into the body, it went ahead digesting tissue all around it, causing severe reactions. A long time ago surgeons devised an ingenious process of sewing the edges of these pancreatic cysts to the edges of the skin wall of an abdominal incision by a process called marsupialization. The operation created something like the pouch of the kangaroo, hence the name.

In cases of excess insulin reaction, however, a peculiar sort of tumor was found, a tumor composed of insulin-producing cells from the islands of Langerhans. These tumors were usually benign; that is, they were not cancers but simply little knobs of tissue like the small fat tumors that appear now and then beneath the skin of anyone. Reasoning that removal of the tumors would result in removing the extra insulin factory, surgeons began to operate on these cases.

Fortunately the location of the tumors makes surgery relatively simple—for the pancreas, that is, where no surgery is simple. The narrow, extended portion of the pancreas, called the tail, where most of those benign adenomas occur, is relatively free and can be approached without much difficulty. The tumor-bearing portion of the organ is removed and the cut end sewn up. The blood sugar returns to normal, the convulsions stop, and the patient no longer has an excuse to eat candy.

Successful attacks on the pancreas, hitherto considered so surgically inaccessible, emboldened surgeons to tackle another problem in this region, one that until then had defied all treatment by the scalpel—carcinoma, the medical name for cancer.

Certain peculiarities of cancer of the pancreas lend themselves to successful surgical attack; others complicate it very much indeed. Cancers of the pancreas grow very slowly and tend to invade other organs only after many months, perhaps even years, of growth. This slowness of growth is the first prerequisite to successful surgical removal of any tumor. However, the inaccessibility of the pancreas would keep surgeons from knowing a tumor was present, but for an anatomical peculiarity.

We have seen in the previous chapter how the common bile duct takes bile from the liver and empties it into the duodenum, the U-shaped first portion of the small intestine. The duct from the pancreas also enters the intestine through the same opening, a pouch-shaped affair called the Ampulla of Vater. In its last inch or so, the pancreatic duct and the common bile duct lie close together; in fact, the bile duct lies against the head of the pancreas, sometimes actually running through the substance of the organ.

Cancer of the pancreas arises almost always in the head of the organ, a bulbous portion lying in the U-shaped crook of the duodenum. This very contiguity of several structures makes possible a warning signal when a cancer of the head of the pancreas begins to grow. Often the tumor is identified long before it has expanded enough to involve other organs or to seed itself out, by the process called metastasis, to other parts of the body.

Briefly, the sequence of events is this. The growing pancreatic tumor presses on the common bile duct, interfering with the passage of bile. The bile begins to back up in the liver, just as it would if a stone were present inside the duct, blocking it. The symptom is the same—jaundice.

Medical students learn very early the significance of jaundice without pain. Stones in the duct usually cause colic, but pressure on the duct from outside causes no colic, therefore no pain. Painless jaundice in a person in the cancer age is strongly suggestive of cancer of the head of the pancreas; often it is the only sign. Usually the gall bladder, if present, will dilate from the back pressure of the bile and may be felt as a sausage-shaped tumor beneath the edge of the ribs on the right side.

Less than twenty years ago the occurrence of this chain of signs and symptoms had only one answer—death. Thanks to the skill and daring of a number of surgeons, led by famed New Yorker, Dr. Allen O. Whipple, many cases can now be saved.

Before Dr. Whipple and other surgeons began the removal of large portions of the pancreas for cancer, surgery had been limited to treatment for relief from the intense discomfort of jaundice. This consisted of an ingenious operation whereby an opening was made between the gall bladder and the small intestine. Bile then poured down from the liver, rebounded from the obstruction to the common bile duct, reversed its way up into the gall bladder, and escaped into the small intestine through the artificial opening. The operation gave relief from the intolerable itching and ever-present danger of hemorrhage to the jaundiced sufferer, but of course exerted no effect on the growth of the cancer.

Removal of the pancreas is a formidable surgical procedure, and is approached with all the care with which a general plans a major campaign. Because of this care and because of the steadily increasing skill of surgeons in this field, more and more cases of pancreatic malignancy are successfully operated on every year.

First in preparation for the operation comes a thorough reconnaissance of the patient's condition, using all the laboratory procedures that have proved their worth in evaluating liver damage. Then follows the usual preoperative preparation—injections of vitamin K, transfusions, and a high protein, carbohydrate, and vitamin intake. All these must be done before the actual operation.

Even with the incision made, with the anesthetist controlling the level of anesthesia by means of a continuous spinal injection or plying a patient with anesthetic gases through a tube in the trachea, the surgeon must decide whether the end justifies the means. He feels the tumor carefully, then searches the tissues on each side for the telltale lumps that mean that lymph glands have already become involved, making operation all but useless. Next he searches the liver carefully, for a tumor nodule in the liver means that metastasis, the seeding out of cancer cells through the blood stream, has already occurred. Knowing the disposition and extent of the enemy, the surgeon is now ready to proceed.

First to be accomplished is a diversion of the flow of bile from the common bile duct, part of which will have to be removed since the tumor presses directly on it. This is sometimes accomplished at a separate operation before the main tumor is attacked. If the gall bladder is present, it is connected to the small intestine. If absent, a much more difficult connection between the cut end of the bile duct and the bowel must be accomplished with meticulous stitching.

The stomach is next cut in two and its upper end connected —surgeons call this an anastomosis—to the small intestine, well below the tumor. The pancreas, the duodenum, and the lower end of the common bile duct are now isolated and can be removed. This is a far from simple procedure, however, for the gland lies directly on the great artery carrying blood to the entire upper digestive tract and close to the great blood-carrying trunks for the whole lower half of the body and legs, the aorta and vena cava. Small wonder, then, that the operation takes hours of meticulous dissection, tying off each tiny blood vessel to prevent hemorrhage. But when a life is at stake, no one begrudges the time spent.

One other thing about the pancreas holds the attention of scientists; the possibility that some day a method may be worked out to graft portions of living pancreatic tissue, with the insulin-producing islands of Langerhans, into the bodies of diabetics, particularly children, who are otherwise doomed to a life of daily insulin injections. A few things seem to point the way toward a solution to the problem, although they may not be said to indicate yet that the answer is even in sight.

The problem involved is one that surgeons have tackled before in the case of burns involving large portions of the body, when they wish to graft skin to tide the sick person over the period of marked general depression that follows severe burns. Skin grafts taken from another person, preferably of the same blood type, often take and grow quite rapidly at first. Then, frequently about two weeks after grafting, the entire foreign skin surface disappears almost overnight, apparently absorbed by the body.

Several years ago a group of researchers started working on the problem of grafting tissue, especially gland tissue, from

ne person to another. Generally speaking, in spite of a lot
of hokum about monkey glands and such, authorities agree
that such homografts (between individuals of the same
species), as distinguished from isografts (from one part of a
person to another part of the same person), do not live. But
suppose the cells to be grafted were allowed to live for a
while in the tissue fluids of the person to whom they were to
be transferred; would it be possible for them to become ac-
customed to the new host and proceed to grow and function
normally?

It is an interesting question, and some results are encouraging. Growth of body cells outside the body is possible by
means of tissue cultures now widely used in studying cancer.
The particular problem with diabetes revolves around removing a portion of pancreas from a normal person at
operation, culturing the island cells in the blood plasma of
the person to receive the graft, and then putting these ac-
climated cells into the recipient's body, where they would,
theoretically at least, grow and produce insulin.

An analogous thing occurs during pregnancy in a diabetic
mother. The child's pancreas produces insulin, which is absorbed into the mother's circulation, usually making her diabetes considerably less severe for the duration of pregnancy,
and incidentally making her liable to a sudden backset after
the child is born.

The chances of survival of such transplanted gland tissue
depend largely on its being grafted into a region with a
plentiful blood supply. One method of doing this is to place
the graft inside a vein, where it is continuously exposed to
the blood, but this procedure is liable to set up clot formation
in the vein, causing possible undesirable side effects. An ingenious experimental placing of grafts of this type was recently described whereby the gland tissue was injected into
the blood stream going to the lungs so it could lodge in the
spongy lung tissue, certainly giving it the richest blood supply
possible anywhere in the body.

With the tremendous advances made in blood-vessel surgery in recent years, a plan once regarded as almost impossible seems much more feasible now. This plan envisions
the removal of an entire pancreas, immediately after death

from accident or other cause, with its tissues and blood vessels intact. These are then connected to those of the host and the organ is set to functioning with this blood supply.

This procedure is not nearly so wild as it sounds. Methods have been devised whereby such blood supply could be connected by means of tiny metal tubes that fit into arteries and veins to carry blood through them past the artificial connections, clotting being prevented by one of the very effective agents such as heparin or dicumarol. The trypsin-forming gland cells would degenerate then and the islands of Langerhans remain to carry on their function of manufacturing insulin.

Experimentally, animal extremities have been amputated, refrigerated for as much as twenty-four hours, then replaced, the blood vessels, muscles, and nerves connected once more, and complete healing has occurred. It is not too fantastic to believe that in the not too far distant future such transplanting of human organs and tissues will be feasible, perhaps commonplace. When it does happen many degenerative diseases, including diabetes, may be eliminated by surgery.

9.

CHEST SURGERY COMES OF AGE

*Surgery and medicine in respiratory infections—
Sucking wounds—Needles and drains—Anesthesia in modern chest surgery—Intratracheal
tubes—Removal of entire lung*

War has a habit of compensating for its evils to a partial
degree, at least, by giving the world new scientific and medical discoveries that might have been years in developing but
for the stimulus of conflict and the multiple technical problems that arise. A classic example of this is radar, a relatively
unimportant laboratory curiosity until it exploded into the
headlines with the disclosure of the near miracles it can
perform in locating enemy submarines and aircraft. Most
startling of all was the atomic bomb and its even more lethal
big brother, the hydrogen bomb.

It is not only in battle wounds that the skill of medical
men turned soldiers is really tried. For with war come numerous other pestilences. Diseases that are normally only occasional occurrences, dependent for their spread on contagion
—which is defeated in civil life by segregation of the populace
into small groups as families—break out with renewed vigor
when men are thrown together in close contact and in large
numbers at army camps. Here more than anywhere are all the
basic ingredients for a witches' brew of contagion.

Medical officers in the armed services labor endlessly to
stay the progress of contagious diseases, such as influenza,
meningitis, scarlet fever, mumps, measles, and perhaps the
greatest cause of time lost, if the least severe, the common
cold. In World War II, preventive medicine was developed to

a high degree. The sulfonamide drugs, taken in small doses daily during an epidemic, such as meningitis, and typhus vaccine are two examples of the devices of mass protection that kept down the spread of contagion.

Even with all their methods of disease prevention and disease-spread control, medical officers aided by members of that group of "Soldiers of the Spray Gun," the Sanitary Corps, were unable to prevent epidemics of respiratory infection—call it grippe, call it influenza, or what you will—from sweeping each winter through the camps and through the country. No one has been able definitely to isolate the virus of these epidemics, to lay a finger on it and say this one was the cause, and what is more important, to destroy it and stop the spread of the disease.

Series of tests have been run on many occasions, with patients coming through clinics and being given alternately sulfa drugs and white pills of the same size. The results have been uniform, even when the antibiotic drugs were substituted for the sulfa compounds. The incidence of colds, the great group of miscellaneous troubles that we label "upper respiratory infections," has not been affected. Perhaps the incidence of complication has been reduced in those who took sulfa or antibiotics; perhaps there were fewer running ears, less pneumonia. Military epidemiologists weren't even sure of that, although civilian study seems to indicate that it is true.

Unfortunately, World War II epidemics were mild in character—unfortunately, that is, for those studying them but certainly not for those affected. Many were affected, but few died. Undoubtedly this was largely due to the vigilance of the Medical Corps, which shoved protesting soldiers into bed at the first sign of fever, thus taking them away from their buddies and stopping the spread of infection while it was still in the early stages. A lot of hospital beds were filled that way, filled with only slightly sick soldiers, but all the evidence goes to prove that this is no false economy. Preventing a respiratory epidemic is a major victory.

We came through wartime winters with nothing resembling a major disaster on the respiratory-disease front. Perhaps we can continue to do so, but the epidemiologists would not give odds on this. Virus infections, such as influenza, sometimes have a habit of building up their virulence as they pass through increasingly large numbers of human hosts. Bacteria often behave the same way; in fact, this passage from host to host is one way of building up and studying the virulence of a particular germ or virus. Will the virus—and even the ultra-electron-microscope has not definitely told us that a virus is anything but an incredibly small germ—of respiratory infection grow in strength and health-damaging potency in the same way?

Nobody knows; we can only wait and see. Vaccines have been developed that seem to hold out some hope of achieving protection against the marauder before it actually attacks the individual. Against some types of respiratory virus it seems definitely to be of value, but there again one cannot always be sure of the enemy that is going to strike a particular person.

As time goes on, undoubtedly, those epidemiologists, those tireless laboratory specialists, those weary officers shooting vaccine into thousands of healthy subjects and then following up by searching through stacks of records to see if resistance to the virus that flies through the air was increased—all of them working together will find the answer and erase those yearly recurring epidemics of cough, fever, and bone ache, just as they have eradicated smallpox, diphtheria, tetanus, typhus, and a host of others by means of vaccines. Poliomyelitis, it seems, will be next to be wiped out.

Considering our inability to control respiratory infection now with all the weapons of military preventive medicine, it is small wonder that doctors' hands were tied in World War I, when the great influenza epidemics appeared, brought by a virus many times more virulent than those that have swept the country in the past decade or so. There's no denying the fact that this influenza virus was the most evil member of the motley, invisible crew ever to attack the human race. Evil and incredibly powerful, leaping apparently unscalable barriers to bring disease to people wherever they were, sometimes appearing even in ships at sea.

Never before had an epidemic spread through the world with such rapidity. Never before had a disease attacked people by hundreds and even thousands overnight, with no way to trace the source.

Never before had simple respiratory infection, if this could be called simple, carried with it such a toll of complications. Patients went rapidly from the early stages of cough, fever, and the shaking ague of bone-splitting pains to the gasping, delirious, dry-skinned picture of influenza pneumonia. By thousands they developed it and by thousands they died.

This was not the type of pneumonia doctors of that time knew so well, the kind that showed fever and toxicity and chests solid with the exudates of inflammation. They'd been treating that kind of pneumonia for years with fomentations, with mustard plasters, with croup tents under which the sick inhaled the pungent aromatic steams that helped to allay the irritation. Often this pneumonia ended with that dramatic "crisis" when the temperature plummeted suddenly to the normal line and remained there while the patient miraculously came back to life. But the influenza pneumonia was a long, dragging kind. The post mortem table showed patchy, grayish areas throughout the lungs, areas that often teemed with the violet-staining, long pearl strands of the streptococcus.

Frequently, too, these patients went into another stage—if they lived through the first one—in which almost normal-sounding chests suddenly lost the resonant quality of breathing lung upon examination and became flat and solid sounding, as if the examining doctor were tapping a container filled with water. And the X-ray showed just about that: a chest filled with fluid.

Doctors had seen fluid develop after the other kind of pneumonia, the kind they called "lobar," and then they knew what to do. They tapped the chest with a needle, and if they found pus, the surgeon took out a little section of rib and made a hole into the chest cavity. They found pus in this new type of pneumonia, too, plenty of pus, but it was different from what they found in the lobar kind. This was very thin; the other was thick. But pus meant empyema to them, and empyema meant surgery.

So the surgeons went to work and started to drain out that pus. They took out sections of ribs and made little windows into the chest cavity just as they had been in the habit of doing. That would take care of everything, they thought; it always had before. Let out the pus and the fever would fall, the patient would rapidly improve.

But what happened this time? Disaster! There was no other name for it.

These cases with the thin pus didn't behave as empyemas should. The pus drained out, it is true, but air rushed in. The little windows were all at once not simple outlets for the inflammation but horrible, sucking, whistling openings. The patients, sick from long assault by the toxins of the streptococcus, didn't stand this added burden very well. Many got worse rapidly; some died. Everywhere the picture was the same, in military life and in civilian life, for the surgeons in making those windows were only following the accepted principles of surgery. It didn't take long to show everybody that their whole idea of chest-pus surgery had to be revised, and some other way found to handle these cases.

An investigating commission of doctors was appointed, leaders in the medical, surgical, laboratory, and teaching fields. They studied the problem from all angles, and when the results were in—fortunately in not too long a time—a new field of surgery was born. What this commission did was to apply to chest surgery what every medical student is taught—physiology, the science of function that delves into every process of the body to see just how it works.

What they found is simple now; every surgery student knows it by heart. But it was a new thing in those days, and it has saved literally thousands of lives since then, not only in case of empyema—for fortunately the widespread use of pneumonia-fighting drugs in our own time has cut the occurrence of empyema to a very low level—but particularly in the handling of chest injuries.

When doctors at the post mortem table looked into the chests of patients who had died from this influenza-following pneumonia, they saw few if any adhesions between the lungs and the inside of the chest. Usually in empyema the lungs stuck fast to the inner wall of the chest, especially around the accumulation of pus, but this time there was little if any sticking. So when the surgeon opened his window into the chest, instead of entering a small area of pus completely walled off from the rest of the chest cavity, what he'd always done before when he operated on an empyema, he was opening directly into the chest cavity itself, letting air between the chest wall and the lung.

Doctors knew already what happened when you put air into the chest around the lungs; they even had a name for it, "pneumothorax," or simply air-in-chest. They had used this method to compress lungs diseased with tuberculosis and had often seen their patients recover miraculously from what had appeared to be a hopeless condition. Air in the chest didn't bother their tubercular patients very much. They could collapse the whole lung without interfering too much with the patient's breathing. What was so different here?

They found the answer to that, too. Injection of air into the chest forms a cushion that pushes the lung down until it is collapsed and remains so. It fills up the chest with air, rather than lung. But that is almost like normal, for the lung is largely air anyway, so spongy is its construction. What is most important, the other lung goes on working to carry on the important function of breathing. It is disturbed but little in that function. And the middle partition in the chest—the great blood vessels and the heart, which make up the middle bulwark separating the lungs that the doctors call the "mediastinum"—isn't disturbed too much, either. This air is closed in the chest, a closed pneumothorax. It isn't dangerous so long as too much air is not injected to embarrass the other lung.

But this other form of air-in-chest, the one with the open window made by the surgeon, was a different matter altogether. Air rushed in and out of the hole with each breathing movement, making a harsh, sucking noise. They could look in that window with a flashlight and see what was happening. Every time air rushed into the chest with inspiration, it pushed the middle layer over; when it ran out again with expiration, the mediastinum flapped back. All that motion interfered with the proper action of the heart, and the pressure of the air in a space where there was normally a partial vacuum, tended to interfere with the flow of blood through the great thin-walled veins to the heart. So they called this "mediastinal flutter."

Here were two reasons, then, why those patients with the

empyemas without adhesions didn't do well. One was the collapse of the lung, which cut the flow of oxygen into the blood stream almost by half. The other was the "flutter," which interfered with the heart action. It looked like enough to explain the whole thing. Now we know that there is another factor more important than either of those two.

A strange thing also happens when one of these open-pneumothorax conditions occurs, whether from the surgeon's operation or from a wound penetrating the chest wall. Normally, air goes in and out through the windpipe and the opening at the larynx called the glottis, which is closed and opened by the vocal cords. That's simple and normal, and it goes on that way, even if one lung is collapsed by air with a closed pneumothorax.

When there's an opening in the chest, however, the story is different. When you breathe in then, the lung on the open side remains collapsed, because opening the chest has released the tiny amount of vacuum that insures that the normal lung will follow the chest wall as it expands in the movement of breathing. Now strain, which means closing the glottis and trying to push air out of the lungs, and what happens? The pressure of straining becomes greater than atmospheric pressure and it blows up the collapsed lung. In other words, the normal lung is exhaling, but the collapsed lung is inhaling. That's what chest surgeons call "paradoxical respiration." Instead of both lungs breathing in and out normally, one breathes in and the other breathes out.

But, and here's the danger, so long as the glottis remains closed and no fresh air enters, the lungs are breathing one from the other, and the oxygen supply of the air shuttled back and forth in this way is soon used up. Unless more oxygen gets in through the glottis, the patient dies from asphyxia, oxygen-lack, in a very short time.

Naturally, a patient suffering from oxygen-lack isn't going to keep his glottis closed. He will be straining to breathe in all the air he can, but that's just what he shouldn't do—strain. Straining raises the pressure in his lungs-windpipe system above atmospheric, and immediately he blows up the collapsed lung, wasting air needlessly again. Along with this he feels his lack of oxygen and is naturally apprehensive, and thus liable to breathe rapidly and gasp for air, thereby making bad matters worse. Too, the presence of air in the sensitive lining pleura of the chest cavity and lung causes him to cough, again increasing the pressure.

All this came out of the researches of the commission to study empyema, or rather they brought to the attention of surgeons everywhere the importance of these facts, which physiologists generally had already known. So surgeons stopped treating these thin-pus empyemas by making cases of open pneumothorax out of them. Instead they put in needles and drew off the pus, until it got thick, until adhesions formed between the two layers of the pleura and walled off the pus, localizing it to one section of the chest. When finally they did make a window, the lung was so stuck to the chest wall that it didn't collapse, and there was no trouble.

Progress was rapid after that; the mortality rate from empyema went down quickly. Ingenious devices were made so that a small tube could be shoved through the muscles between the ribs, maintaining an airtight fit around the tube and allowing the pus to be drawn off without frequent needlings. To this was added a system of irrigation by which antiseptic fluid could flow gently in and out through the tube, washing out the pus and healing up the inflamed pleura at the same time the lung was expanding into the space formerly occupied by the empyema.

A simple set of principles had been worked out now to treat empyema, whether the ordinary thick-pus kind or the streptococcic kind. Once the lung was stuck to the chest wall, you could open with freedom. But that was the least important product of this new knowledge of chest physiology and its application to healing disease.

Surgeons had long wished to tackle diseases inside the chest, inside the lung, even inside the heart. But always there had been the difficulty of an open pneumothorax. They knew that as long as the patient breathed quietly under the anesthetic, as long as he didn't cough or strain, they could open the chest and could work around the vital heart and lungs without danger. In fact, various kinds of special pressure chambers had been devised so that operations could be carried on inside them and the lung-pressure relationships kept normal during the procedure. But most of them were too bulky and unhandy for general use.

What they needed was some way of taking care of the patient's breathing and his chest-pressure relationships under all conditions. Obviously the answer was some method of keeping the airway to the lung open and pumping oxygen along with the anesthetic gases directly into the lung under slightly increased pressure. In that way the good lung could be kept breathing normally while the surgeon opened the chest and took his time about operating on the other side.

It didn't take the anesthetists long to figure that one out. Doctors had for a long time been inserting slender metal tubes with lights on them into the windpipe and bronchial passages of children who had inhaled safety pins or other foreign bodies into their lungs. It was dangerous and difficult to keep a metal tube in for the hours sometimes needed for a major chest operation, but there was no reason why a rubber tube wouldn't do the same thing.

And so they started using intratracheal tubes, some with tiny balloons around the lower end so that an airtight fit could be obtained between the tube and the windpipe. The expert anesthetist puts the patient to sleep in the ordinary way. Then he takes a short instrument with a light on the end, called a laryngoscope, inserts it into the back of the throat, and locates the opening into the windpipe. Next he slips a soft rubber tube directly into the windpipe, establishing a free airway to the lung. To this he connects his anesthetic machine, and everything is ready. Even if both chest cavities are accidentally opened, the anesthetist can inflate the lungs regularly by squeezing the breathing bag on his anesthetic machine. The surgeon is free to do whatever is necessary, to remove a lung for cancer, to sew up a wound of the heart, or open a closed heart valve. He works unhurriedly, unworried about the breathing of the patient.

And so we have another example of how one calamity brings about a new knowledge that helps avert or at least nullify many of the ill effects of another. Those things learned in World War I empyema cases saved lives by the thousands in World War II. Many a soldier in World War I lay gasping on the field, slowly dying while the horrible whistling sound of his open chest wound pounded at his ears. Medical soldiers, aid-station doctors, tried to help, but they did not know how to combat this form of suffocation.

Now the procedure is simple. Every enlisted man—not just the medical soldiers but every soldier—is shown a film strip or a moving picture telling him the basic facts about first aid. One thing is stressed time and time again; sucking wounds, accidental cases of open pneumothorax, in which the whistling in-and-out flow of air can be heard, must be closed by whatever method can be found; a dressing, a handkerchief, whatever is available, must be placed over the wound and pressure applied until no air can flow in and out.

Once a dressing covers the wound and pressure is maintained, the open pneumothorax is immediately converted into a closed one; the normal lung is now able to breathe properly, without shuttling its air back and forth in the fruitless process of "paradoxical respiration." The first person to reach the wounded soldier, or the soldier himself, applies the pressure, and it must never be released until the casualty is back at the hospital, where the wound can be closed. The medical soldiers carry a bulky dressing for just this purpose, and they are trained until they are adept at applying this stopgap to control lung collapse. Then they wait or see that the casualty is watched until other medical personnel can come to take him to the rear.

At the hospital, chest wounds are given a priority, as are those of the abdominal cavity. Here the wound is excised, for if foreign bodies get into the wound, muscle loses its blood supply and infection can develop just as in any other wound, carrying with it danger of involvement of the lung. The anesthetist will have a portable anesthetic machine, with intratracheal tubes to use if needed.

The surgeon *débrides* the wound, removes foreign bodies lying close at hand, treats it very much as he would any other wound. He doesn't waste time digging into a lung for a piece of shrapnel, for he knows it is safer to remove that later, if it becomes necessary at all. Then he closes the opening in the chest wall in one of several ways, by sewing it directly together, often impossible, or more frequently by sewing a flap of muscle from the muscular wall of the chest.

Before he places the final suture, the surgeon often takes a small rubber tube and inserts it between the ribs below the wound, so as to drain out blood and air from the chest as it accumulates. But he clamps it tightly so that no air can enter through this drainage tube, or better still, attaches it to a simple valve mechanism. This done, he leaves the outer wound open and gives the patient heavy doses of penicillin or the other antibiotic drugs. He knows that these bulwarks against the spread of infection will do more than anything to keep any inflammation that may occur from getting into the body and poisoning it with the toxins of septicemia.

Modern chest surgeons know how to handle war-time injuries, from the front line all the way back to the great chest centers in this country where complicated cases are finally cured. Here delicate plastic operations are performed to collapse areas where bullets and infections have destroyed sections of the lung, and foreign bodies causing troublesome symptoms are removed by specialists who devote their entire life work to this very special field. But the real test is at the front, in the application by the soldier or by his medical-corps buddy of the cumulative knowledge of chest physiology, in the simple form of a bulky dressing that changes an open pneumothorax to a closed one.

Many cases have no open wound, yet carry with them just as much danger as the dramatic open pneumothorax. These constitute another group of air-in-chest injuries, called tension pneumothorax, perhaps the most common of chest injuries in civil life. What happens is that a bullet or a knife penetrates the chest wall and goes into the lung. The chest-wall opening is quickly closed by contraction of the muscles, but the lung keeps pumping air into the chest through the valvelike opening into its substance made by the missile. With inspiration the lung valve closes; with expiration it pumps out more air. This air is trapped in the chest, and the pressure steadily increases with each breathing movement. Soon, unless something is done, the normal lung is also collapsed by the pressure and the patient suffocates.

The treatment of tension pneumothorax is simple, but it must be administered at once. A needle is thrust into the injured side of the chest, allowing an escape for the air being pumped out. The needle is so small that very little air enters the chest through it, but it acts as a sort of pop-off valve to prevent too much pressure from accumulating in the chest. Then a tube is attached to the needle and carried down to the floor, where it is placed in a bottle of water. Air now bubbles out through the water, but none can enter the tube. In this way a simple and effective valve is made.

Often in these puncture injuries of the chest, blood accumulates in large quantities along with the air. The pressure of air and blood will usually stop both hemorrhage and escape of air, and doctors often leave these cases strictly alone and see both air and blood absorb rapidly. In many cases, however, the blood clots inside the chest, and unless the surgeon is alert to recognize this complication, much time may be lost in recovery. Failure of blood in the chest to absorb quickly is treated by opening it, evacuating the clotted blood and allowing the lung to expand. In war wounds of the chest particularly, this simple operation has proved of great value.

The application of simple physical and physiological scientific principles has opened up two new worlds to the surgeon. Not only can he now work with impunity on the lungs, but the heart itself has been brought within the domain of surgery, crossing the last frontier.

10.

HEART SURGERY

*The inside of the heart—Thrombosis and he-
parin in heart surgery—Dicoumarin—Cardiac
tamponade—Sewing up a heart wound—Pericarditis in pneumonia and rheumatic infection—
Removing the heart's cover—Congenital heart
disease in children—Hypothermia—Heart-valve
surgery*

When surgeons began to look to surgery's last remaining
frontier, the heart, they found a lot of the preliminary work
already accomplished. Tackling the heart surgically means
opening the chest of course, but positive-pressure anesthesia
already had made long operations in the open chest possible.
Another problem was clotting of the blood, called thrombosis,
which occurs wherever a blood vessel is damaged by whatever agent, a bullet or a surgeon's knife. Thrombosis tends to
close up the vessel at this point. Worse still, pieces of it break
off and travel in the blood stream, causing often fatal emboli
to the lungs and brain.

That problem was largely solved with heparin, the clot-
preventing substance. Isolated chemically and now prepared
for medical use so that it can be injected into the circulation
in intermittent or continuous doses, heparin decreases the clotting power of the blood to a remarkable degree, preventing
the formation of thrombi where blood vessels are connected
together by surgical operation, or where a great artery is
opened to remove the clot that may suddenly shut off the
blood supply to an entire leg of a heart patient. It was a

wonderful discovery, one destined to revolutionize the lusty science of blood-vessel surgery.

As if heparin weren't enough of an accomplishment, along came another group of scientists, studying the peculiar disease animals get after eating large quantities of sweet clover, a disease in which they hemorrhage into their own tissues and body cavities and often die. This group reasoned that there was in this sweet clover a substance that acted like heparin, but unlike heparin, could be eaten and still do its work. Eat heparin and the stomach digests it immediately, ending its clot-preventing power. But the clover substance withstands digestive action, as witness the fact that it works after being eaten in clover by the animal. From these researchers came Dicoumarin, which does the same thing as heparin and can be taken by mouth besides, just as you'd take an aspirin or a dose of soda.

Meanwhile other surgeons had already tackled the heart, but they hadn't done it as a matter of election. They'd done it as an emergency, to save lives. For civilians don't wait for wars to carry on their own little private conflicts. Some sections of the country are worse than others, of course, and stabbing between the ribs with long, slender knives is a fairly common practice in some areas. Usually this habit doesn't produce very bad results. The knife goes into the lung as a rule, there is an escape of air and blood into the chest, and the collapse of the lung by the air stops the bleeding and escape of air into the pleura cavity. The patient has a little shortness of breath for a day or so, and maybe a little fever, but the whole thing is absorbed, and nothing happens. Every surgeon in a large city hospital has seen dozens and even hundreds of such cases.

But every now and then the wound moves closer to the center of the chest and then there is real trouble. This time the knife, or sometimes a bullet, even an ice pick, enters the heart, and blood spurts through the opening with each beat of the heart. Usually the hemorrhage doesn't appear through the wound that enters the skin, for as in the case of the wound in the lung, the chest muscles tend to close that opening. What happens is that blood pours out into the tough bag, called the pericardium, that surrounds the heart. As it fills the bag, something has to give way. Usually this is the thing that can least afford to be disturbed in its function, the heart. Pressure of blood in the pericardium gradually decreases the space in which the heart can beat and squeezes it, just as one might squeeze it with one's own hand.

Doctors call this squeezing process "cardiac tamponade," which means simply an increased pressure on the heart exerted by the blood it is pumping out through the opening in the heart wall. Tamponade is an emergency that calls for immediate action, or death will ensue at once. Rarely does such an injury occur in a place where the patient can be rushed immediately to an operating room set up and ready for a heart operation. There has to be a period of getting the patient to the hospital, making the diagnosis, and getting him to the operating room. In that time he may very well die unless the emergency is recognized and tackled courageously at once.

Staffs of great city hospitals are trained in this matter of heart wounds, trained to recognize from the thready or absent pulse, the distant heart sounds in the stethoscope, the absence of heart movement when the chest is examined with the fluoroscope, the picture of cardiac tamponade. And they get to work at once, with a syringe and a needle, to remove from the pericardium some of the blood pressing upon the heart.

At first all these patients were operated on as soon as an operating room could be prepared, but before long it was discovered that removing the blood from the pericardium by repeated insertions of a needle if necessary often allowed the heart wound to close itself up without surgery. Now, large series of cases have been reported in which only a few actually needed operation. Most of them were taken care of simply by removing the blood from the pericardial sac, allowing the heart to beat and letting nature seal the wound in the heart muscle through clotting.

Some cases, of course, still require actual surgery, but there is nothing particularly difficult about sewing up a heart wound. The most important work has been done by the resident or intern who kept the patient alive by removing blood from the pericardium. During the operation a couple of rib ends are removed from the front of the chest wall to expose the heart. A suture is usually put through the tip of the heart, the apex, and used as a guy while the wound itself is closed with a few quick strands of silk. There usually isn't much difficulty in this either, for the heart, being thick and muscular, holds stitches well. That also accounts for the fact that these wounds often close themselves.

When World War II came along, the groundwork in treating heart injuries had already been done. War wounds of the heart do not often come to treatment in even the front-line hospitals, however. Bullet and shrapnel wounds in this area are much more likely to be fatal than the knife wounds of civilian combat, but if they do reach the operating rooms, the surgical principles for handling them are clear. Every war surgeon was familiar with them and could put them into application at once, and many lives were undoubtedly saved because of that knowledge.

Another serious problem in heart surgery was, and still is, pericarditis. In some diseases, such as severe pneumonia, rheumatic infection, or almost any severe streptococcus infection, the sac surrounding the heart may become infected also, usually by way of the blood stream, in which, we now know, bacteria travel in large numbers during almost any severe disease caused by micro-organisms. The tough pericardial sac then fills up with pus, and the effect is very much the same as if it were filled with blood. Pressure interferes with the heart action, adding that burden to a body already in trouble from a severe infection.

Surgeons have long known that in pericarditis cases they can make a small window through the lower front portion of the chest and allow this pus to drain out, relieving the pressure and allowing the heart room to work. Irrigations, too, can be carried out through this window, decreasing the likelihood of adhesions between the pericardium and the heart, which may later interfere with the operation of that vital blood pump.

A less conspicuous, more chronic inflammation of the pericardium leaves it thick and tough, sometimes plastered tightly around the heart. This chronic form of pericarditis gradually constricts the heart's action until the circulation can no longer be kept up properly, and the patient begins to show definite signs that the blood isn't being pumped efficiently. These signs are fluid in the abdomen, conspicuous dilation of veins of the skin, evidence of oxygen-lack, moisture in the lungs; all mean impending heart failure.

Surgeons long ago began to study these cases, many of them children doomed to an early death unless the condition was relieved. They used their trained senses to tell them what had happened, but they didn't stop at that. It wasn't right to subject a patient to an operation of such magnitude as would be required unless you could be sure of what had happened. So they took advantage of a peculiarity of the heart. Move around, turn from one side to another, and the normal heart moves also, shifting slightly in position with each change. Then take an electrocardiogram—the electric heart picture that tells exactly what is going on in the muscle of the heart—and the picture is slightly different in each position. Cardiologists call that a shift of the "electrical axis" of the heart. Such a shift is perfectly normal.

With the heart sealed into position by a chronically inflamed, leathery pericardium, however, a heart so small and contracted that it is unable to do its work efficiently, there is a different picture. The heart cannot shift with movement so the electrocardiogram is the same in all positions, because the electrical axis of the heart doesn't move. That's the clinching fact in this diagnosis of chronic constrictive pericarditis.

Once the diagnosis is established, the surgeon can tackle the problem with certainty. He makes an incision through the chest, exposing the heart, and goes about the business of removing the whole front of the leathery pericardium. Sometimes he even has to separate it from the surface of the heart, peeling it away. But he keeps on until the heart is free to expand and beat normally. After this operation, a dramatic thing usually happens. Since the heart can do its work now, the shortness of breath disappears, the color returns to normal, the fluid in the body cavities is absorbed, and the veins lose their distended appearance.

For obvious reasons, the heart does not lend itself easily to surgical procedures that involve either opening the organ or opening the large blood vessels nearby. Operating on the heart is like trying to repair an engine while the engine is running. This engine, of course, must be kept running throughout the operation if the patient is to stay alive. In surgery of the heart there is the danger of stopping the engine, of fatal bleeding; above all there is the dangerous fact that any damage to the interior of the blood-vessel system is usually followed by the formation of clots, either stationary (thrombi) or floating (emboli), which may block the circulation.

Essentially the heart is a double-chambered, muscle-powered pump. With each beat this pump drives blood through the circulatory system. The cycle begins when blood returning from the body tissues comes by way of the great veins into the right auricle of the heart. It passes then through a set of valves into the right ventricle. From there the heartbeat pumps the blood through the pulmonary arteries into the lungs, where it takes up oxygen.

The oxygenated blood, returning to the heart through the pulmonary veins, enters the left auricle, passes on to the left ventricle and then, by the powerful systolic contraction of the heart, is pumped under considerable pressure out to the tiniest arteries, carrying food and oxygen to all the body cells. After giving up some of its oxygen and taking carbon dioxide and other waste products from the tissues, the blood then returns to the heart through the veins. The heart, lying between the lungs and surrounded by the pericardium, is in intimate contact with both lungs and the pleura.

The field of the most striking advances in heart surgery in the last two decades is the large category of disorders arising from congenital defects of the heart. Many children are born with one or more of the chambers or valves missing, with abnormalities of the valves or arteries that block the free passage of blood, with abnormally developed vessels that cause the flow of blood to by-pass the lungs so it cannot be oxygenated properly, or with defects inside the chambers of the heart, abnormal openings that interfere with the proper flow of blood.

One of the most frequent of the congenital disturbances of the heart has its origin in the failure of the fetus to get rid of a convenient mechanism that becomes most inconvenient after birth. Before birth the fetus, of course, does not need to circulate blood through its lungs; its blood is oxygenated in its mother's circulation. The fetal blood therefore by-passes its uninflated lungs through an ingenious shortcut called the *ductus arteriosus*. This is a short, narrow vessel that carries the blood directly from the pulmonary artery, which goes to the lungs, to the aorta, the great artery through which blood is distributed to most of the body.

When the baby is born and begins to breathe, normally the ductus arteriosus closes and the blood at once begins to circulate through the lungs. In some children, however, the ductus arteriosus fails to close and much of the blood that should go to the lungs is short-circuited through the open vessel.

If the ductus opening is small, so that relatively little blood by-passes the lungs, the child may show few or no ill effects. But if it is large, the youngster soon exhibits certain typical symptoms: low resistance, quick exhaustion after any physical effort, susceptibility to respiratory infection such as bronchopneumonia, and most particularly, the development of the serious disease called subacute bacterial endocarditis, a grave inflammation of the inner lining of the heart and its valves. Most victims of "patent (open) ductus arteriosus" once were doomed to die, either of bacterial endocarditis or of progressive weakening of a heart overloaded by attempting to pump blood faster to obtain more oxygen.

Here again the solution required boldness and skill. It was obvious that the condition could be corrected simply by ligating (tying up) the open passage. But the ductus arteriosus is so intimately connected with the vital aorta and pulmonary artery that surgeons long considered such an operation impossible. In 1938 the Boston surgeon Robert E. Gross finally performed it successfully. His operation was one of the great milestones of heart surgery.

Soon afterward a New York surgeon, Arthur S. W. Touroff, showed that ligation of the patent ductus could cure even those victims who had already contracted subacute bacterial endocarditis—the first cure of what had previously been considered an inevitably fatal disease. Later it was found that penicillin also could clear up subacute bacterial endocarditis, and deaths from this disease now are rare. The operation for patent ductus today is so safe and so successful in skilled hands—the mortality rate is five per cent or less—that pediatricians do not hesitate to recommend it.

The famous "blue-baby" operation pioneered by Dr. Alfred Blalock and Dr. Helen A. Taussig, of Johns Hopkins, is the direct opposite of this operation—a "ductus-in-reverse." The basic result to be achieved—correction of an interference with proper oxygenation of the blood—is the same, but the method is different. In this case the operation involves creating an artificial connection between the lung arteries and the branch of the aorta.

The abnormality that causes the trouble is not a single defect but a curious combination of deformities known as the "tetralogy of Fallot." This quartet of anomalies, which somehow are congenitally linked, was first noticed by the British anatomist William Hunter at the end of the eighteenth century and later described more fully by the nineteenth-century French physician Etienne-Louis Arthur Fallot.

The deformities are: (1) a narrowing of the opening from the heart to the pulmonary arteries, (2) a displacement of the aorta far to the right of its normal position, which constricts both the aorta and the pulmonary arteries, (3) a defect in the wall between the right and left ventricles, which permits blood in one chamber to mix with that of the other, (4) a considerable thickening of the right ventricle.

The net result of this combination of defects is that circulation to the lungs is impaired and mixed venous and arterial blood from the ventricles is pumped into the general circulation, largely by-passing the lungs. It produces a set of markedly characteristic symptoms: cyanosis (blueness of the skin due to lack of sufficient oxygen in the blood); an increase in the number of red blood cells, manufactured by the body in an attempt to compensate for the lowered oxygen supply; clubbed fingers; shortness of breath during even mild exertion; and a rather striking tendency of affected children to squat suddenly on their haunches after exertion in order to rest.

The conquest of this fatal disorder was achieved by a combination of the diagnostic insight of heart specialist Taussig and the surgical skill and daring of surgeon Blalock. It was Dr. Taussig who first proved that the baneful effects of the tetralogy of Fallot were due fundamentally to its interference with the flow of blood to the lungs. The two physicians at once saw that they might save these doomed children by a surgical operation on the arteries to increase the blood flow to the pulmonary system.

Dr. Blalock, who had long been interested in surgery of the great blood vessels, had worked out techniques for changing the connections of these vessels. In experiments on animals he had developed a method whereby he could cut the subclavian artery, which carries blood to the arm and shoulder, and by a procedure called anastomosis attach the stump of this artery to the side of the pulmonary artery going to the lungs. This maneuver shunted the mixed arterial and venous blood that came from the heart back into the lungs, thereby increasing the blood's oxygen supply. Fortunately, the auxiliary circulation to the arm is sufficient to maintain an adequate blood supply to the arm even when the subclavian artery is cut, so severing this channel is not dangerous.

Another difficulty about the operation also was overcome: it was feared that shutting off the blood supply to a lung for a period necessary to make an anastomosis would be dangerous for these already cyanotic patients, but with modern methods of anesthesia this fear has proved unfounded; the oxygen administered during anesthesia actually raises the oxygen level in the blood.

After trying his surgical procedures over and over again in experimental animals, Dr. Blalock performed the first operation on a human in 1945. The success of this operation is now a matter of surgical history. Hundreds of selected cases have been operated on, with a mortality rate less than 10 per cent. The operation has steadily been improved. Blalock himself has varied his technique to fit particular conditions, and the Chicago heart surgeon, Dr. Willis J. Potts, worked out an important modification. He devised an ingenious clamp that closes off a small section of an artery, permitting the surgeon to operate on this section while blood continues to flow through the main channel. With this technique it is possible to anastomose the pulmonary artery directly to the aorta, obviating the need to sever the subclavian artery.

Still another congenital heart condition in which surgery once seemed impossible has yielded to the scalpel. This is coarctation (a narrowing of the aorta), which sharply reduces the flow of blood to the body. In 1944 Dr. Clarence Crawford, surgeon-in-chief of the Surgical Clinic in Stockholm, cut out the narrowed portion of the aorta in such a patient and successfully anastomosed the cut ends together again, thus restoring the free flow of blood. Shortly afterward the Boston surgeon Dr. Robert E. Gross, originator of the patent ductus operation, independently performed a procedure like Crawford's, adding this accomplishment to his already impressive list. Many other cases have been reported since then, including a resection of aneurysms of the aorta, a sacular dilatation of this great artery which is often fatal if not treated surgically.

In the past several years, daring heart surgeons have been able to report the successful closure of defects in the septum of the heart, the partition that separates the right side of the heart from the left. This operation necessitated actual opening of the heart and working inside its cavities. To obtain a bloodless field where the surgeon can see what he is doing, it is necessary to entirely shut off the flow of blood for brief periods. This, however, always poses a considerable danger to the brain, which cannot stand any long absence of an adequate blood supply. At first there seemed no answer to this problem, but quite recently one has been worked out that does increase remarkably the time limit for shutting off the circulation to the brain.

Briefly, this procedure consists of lowering the body temperature and thus lowering the metabolism of the cells so that they do not need nearly so much oxygen as under normal conditions. Called hypothermia, this method of anesthesia is a delicate one, requiring expert knowledge. Generally the temperature lowering is accomplished by one of two methods. In one, the patient is immersed in ice water until the temperature is lowered to the desired level. In the other, he is wrapped in a blanket through which circulates a network of small tubes containing a constant flow of ice water. When the temperature is lowered to the desired level, the flow of the ice water is stopped and the blanket is left beneath the patient during the operation.

Still another method of shutting off the patient's circulation to work inside the heart has been developed very recently, but is used in only a few cases. This ingenious device utilizes the circulation of another person, most commonly a parent of the child being operated upon. It lets the normal person's heart take over for a short time in place of the defective heart pump. Only a very few such cases have been reported, but in certain instances it does seem to offer a definite lifesaving weapon to heart surgery.

Thus surgery has made great strides in three of the four categories of heart disorders—wounds, infections, and congenital abnormalities. A fourth category is the extremely dangerous group of disturbances involving interference of the blood circulation to the heart muscle, such as occurs in coronary thrombosis. Coronary heart disease may result in sudden death or grave weakening of the heart muscle. It remains one of the great challenges to medicine, although a great deal of progress has been made in treating it, notably by use of the anticlotting agents, oxygen, and general supportive therapy.

A coronary attack may come without warning, but fortunately it is sometimes heralded by painful symptoms like those of angina pectoris, which give notice of a failing heart circulation before an actual block of the arteries takes place. With this warning, a fatal break in the coronary blood supply is sometimes avoidable by an operation that improves the blood flow to the damaged heart.

A pioneer in this field of surgery is Dr. Claude Beck, professor of surgery at the Western Reserve Medical School. Dr. Beck has for many years been working on a number of different operations to increase the circulation to the heart muscle where the coronary supply has been damaged. One of the most successful of these utilizes the effect on the heart of an irritating substance placed in the pericardium, the most commonly used agent being talcum powder. There is thus set up a mild irritation that causes adhesions between the heart and the tissues surrounding it, through which a new blood supply may grow into the heart. Dr. Beck and other experimenters have also grafted flaps of muscle from the chest wall to the heart, so that new blood vessels could grow into the damaged organ. In one remarkable case, described in the first chapter, he actually put a patch on a weakened heart wall to avoid the dangerous aneurysm of the heart, which often causes sudden death.

An ingenious approach to this problem has been devised by Montreal surgeon Mercier Fauteux. His operations are designed to increase the flow of blood through the coronary arteries and to slow the flow through the veins coming from the heart. He achieves the former by severing the sympathetic nerves that control constriction of the arteries, thus eliminating such constrictions. He slows the flow in the veins by tying them off at the place where they come together to form the large vessel called the coronary sinus.

As a result of the slowing circulation, the blood stays in contact with the heart muscle longer and is able to transmit more oxygen to it. Undoubtedly as experience with heart and blood-vessel surgery expands, more effective ways of taking care of this number-one killer now will be found, adding still further contributions to the battle against death.

For many, many years one of the greatest unsolved problems in heart surgery was repair of the damage to the heart valves, such as occurs in rheumatic heart disease. Aside from all the other perils that attend operations within the heart—hemorrhage, clotting, fibrillation (disorganization of the rhythm), and stopping of the heart—operations on the delicate valves tend, if not done properly, to create scars that may destroy the beneficial effects of the operation.

Interestingly enough, the first real contribution to this particular type of surgery was made by Dr. Horace G. Smithy, of Charleston, South Carolina, who himself died of rheumatic heart disease before his own operation could be developed to the point where it could save him.

Working with the Smithy technique, many surgeons now have tackled the heart valves themselves. Generally speaking, the operations follow a certain pattern, namely an approach to the interior of the heart through the thin-walled auricular appendage, a small sac that connects with the auricles and through which an incision can be made without a major loss of blood. Briefly, the technique consists of applying a purse-string suture—similar to the type of looped thread that closed the old-fashioned tobacco bag—and opening into the heart within the loop of this suture. Then the surgeon's finger, with a small and ingenious knife blade strapped to it if desired, can be inserted through the opening and the suture drawn tight around his gloved finger to prevent blood loss while he manipulates the finger inside the heart chambers either to dilate the scarred valves or actually to cut through them.

One difficulty in heart surgery, namely the entry of air into the heart whenever it must be opened for any period of time, has been gotten around very ingeniously through the simple expedient of filling the entire heart with salt solution at the end of an operation. Flooding the area around it to remove air allows the closure of whatever wounds have been made in this pool of salt solution while the heart begins to act normally once more and restore the normal circulation. In this way the pumping of air around through the circulation, a dangerous thing particularly to the brain cells, is avoided.

It is safe to say that in the past decade no branch of surgery has shown such amazing progress as heart surgery. With this frontier pushed further and further back almost daily, even more startling progress will undoubtedly be made in the not too distant future. Here again science and surgery have worked together and will continue to accomplish another miracle of modern surgical progress.

AUTHOR'S NOTE: Portions of this chapter appeared in *Scientific American* and are used with the permission of the publishers.

11.

SAVING LIMBS WITH SURGERY

Vascular surgery, one of the greatest contributions of war to peacetime medicine—The circulatory system and the autonomic nervous system—Severance of major blood vessels no longer means amputation—Vitallium splints for injured blood vessels—Pulsating hematoma and aneurysm—New, drastic operations

No one can be certain just what was the greatest peacetime contribution of World War II. It may have been the newer knowledge and interest in tropical medicine so important in Pacific theaters, where every wounded man was considered, and usually found, to have malaria. Or again it may have been the proof that blood transfusions and blood-plasma injections can do miracles in preventing and treating shock from severe wounds. These are important contributions, and there are many others almost equally so, but it seems probable that the greatest new specialty, one that will develop now to its rightful place along with orthopedics, chest surgery, neurosurgery, and general surgery, is vascular surgery, the study and treatment of injuries and diseases involving the circulatory system, the blood vessels of the body.

The circulatory system is a giant network of channels through which blood is pumped everywhere in the body, bringing the vital fluid with its cargo of food, minerals, and other important chemicals. Oxygen, without which body cells cannot live long, is carried by the disc-shaped red blood cells and their cargo of hemoglobin. Interference with the blood supply to the body cells for a few seconds causes oxygen-

116

lack, the blue color of cyanosis shows in the skin, and death occurs in a short time.

Some cells can withstand oxygen-lack for much shorter periods than others. A brain cell may die in a few seconds when its vital oxygen supply is interfered with, while a tissue cell in the toe may live almost indefinitely, under certain conditions, with a small percentage of its normal supply of oxygen. Diseases and injuries involving the circulatory or vascular system are immediate threats to the life of the body as a whole, as well as to the immediate sections involved.

Blood is pumped by the heart through two circuits. The first is the "pulmonary," or lung circuit, where oxygen inhaled from the air is absorbed into the blood and by chemical change into the hemoglobin of the red blood cells, giving the characteristic bright-red color of blood coming from the lungs. The second circuit is the "systemic," by way of the greatest artery, the aorta, and outward through successively smaller channels to end in the vast microscopic-sized capillary network, which surrounds every cell and is known generally as the peripheral vascular bed. Blood passing through the capillary bed enters the veins and by successively larger channels finally makes its way back to the heart to begin once more its circuit of the lungs.

Arteries are thick-walled, elastic, and contain blood under high pressure, hence the spurting flow from a severed artery. Veins are thin-walled and blood is pumped through them largely by the sucking action of the negative pressure created in the chest by the movements of breathing and the pumping action of the muscles lying alongside the veins. Large vessels of the body usually lie side by side, the artery by the vein, with blood flowing in opposite directions in each. Injuries involving arteries almost always involve veins, and sometimes blood flows immediately from the area of high pressure in the arteries to the low pressure of the veins. A communication can then develop, an abnormal connection called an "arteriovenous fistula." These abnormalities constitute the most fascinating and difficult problems for the vascular surgeon.

Fortunately, blood channels are rarely singular; almost always there are branching connections called anastomoses, whereby blood can be shunted around a damaged circuit, much as trains are routed around a temporarily damaged track. These are called collateral channels; without them there would be no vascular surgery, for an injury to the main artery of a limb would mean instant death of the entire limb.

Nor is the size of any artery ever constant over a very long period of time. The needs of the body for blood vary with different sections at different times. Eat a large meal and you need reinforcement in the secondary circuits involving the abdominal organs. Therefore, blood is immediately shunted from the brain and other organs and, as a result, mental work is interfered with during the height of the digestive period.

This shunt is accomplished by an amazingly efficient hair-trigger control system called the autonomic nervous system. It is called autonomic because it is completely automatic; it functions to control our blood needs, as well as many other vital functions, with no conscious effort on our part. It lies in a chain of small nodular accumulations of nervous tissue alongside the spinal cord, connected to it by smaller roots called rami.

Generally these nodes, or ganglia, as they are called, belong to one of two groups, the sympathetic or the parasympathetic system. The two send connections to practically every organ of the body, maintaining a balance on every vital function. Control of size of arteries is maintained by the network of nerve fibers from both systems, which runs in the walls of all the blood vessels. The sympathetic system causes constriction of the arteries, called the vasoconstrictor effect; the parasympathetic causes dilatation, the vasodilator effect. Thus, if blood is needed by the abdominal organs, the mesenteric arteries, which go to the intestinal tract, are dilated, while others are constricted.

A knowledge of these things is essential for the surgeon who handles injuries involving the arteries and the veins. On the early and intelligent treatment of damage to the large blood vessels depends the saving of many limbs. That is why the simple principles of vascular surgery are preached to every embryo surgeon in the course of his training.

In World War I severance of a major blood vessel called for amputation; in World War II it was merely a challenge to the ingenuity of the vascular surgeon. Sixty-five per cent of all war wounds involve the extremities, the leg being affected about twice as frequently as the arm. It is on the treatment of these injuries that the vascular surgeon concentrates his attention.

A bullet into one of the great blood vessels of the abdomen, chest, or to a lesser extent the neck, usually means death from hemorrhage. A bullet into one or more blood vessels of the limbs, properly handled with a tourniquet to control bleeding applied just above the wound, or with a pressure dressing if arteries are not involved, may result in some of the most bizarre surgical pictures imaginable, but nine chances out of ten the limb will be saved.

When an artery is injured without being severed a peculiar sequence of events occurs. The body reacts immediately to cut down the flow of blood to the damaged area. Perhaps this is a normal insult reaction; perhaps it is an intelligent move by the autonomic nervous system to put as little blood as possible through an area that may blow open at any moment. Whatever it is, there is an immediate and widespread constriction of the arteries in that locality known as "vasospasm." To a certain extent this can be considered a protective reaction, but usually it tends to get out of hand. The circulation of the extremity is interfered with, the collateral channels that would normally by-pass the injured area are also shut down, and the limb turns white, showing very much the same effect as having a tourniquet put upon it. If not controlled, this vasospasm may mean gangrene and death of the limb. Fortunately, it is not hard to tip the balance against the spasm and in favor of the dilating effect.

To relieve blood-vessel spasm, novocain—and sometimes later alcohol if the effect is to be prolonged—is injected into the portion of the sympathetic system, the vasoconstrictor nerves, that controls the size of the limb vessels. For the leg, these ganglia are located alongside the spine in the lower back, the lumbar region. For the arm, they are in a similar position in the lower neck and upper chest. They can be reached accurately with long needles, and injections block them effectively. Knocking out the constrictor fibers leaves the dilator fibers in full sway; the vessels resume something like their normal size and blood once more can flow. If there is need for a permanent dilatation of the vessels—and this is notably true in some medical diseases of the blood vessels such as Raynaud's disease, characterized by cold fingers—these ganglia can actually be removed by a relatively simple operation.

When an artery or an artery and vein are severed, a much more difficult situation develops. Strangely enough it is much more dangerous for the injured person if there is merely a hole in the side of the artery than if the vessel is completely cut across. Sever an artery completely and the inner layer, the intima, retracts and draws inward, the muscular layer just outside it contracts, and almost immediately the opening is decreased in size. Often it is closed off entirely and bleeding stops. But tear a hole in the side of the channel and blood pours out with no control, escaping outward if there is an open wound or accumulating in the deeper tissues if there is a small wound of entrance, such as that made by a bullet. Pressure of the blood filling the tissues tends to block vessels, particularly the smaller channels which are badly needed now. This, coupled with the vasospasm that also occurs, places the limb in grave jeopardy. Surgery here is imperative, and skillful surgery is at a premium. The opening in the vessel must be located and controlled quickly.

Rarely in war surgery is it possible to repair the vessel. In a well-equipped surgical center, with tiny vitallium tubes to use as splints—perhaps lined with sections of nearby veins removed for the purpose—and injections of heparin or doses of the sweet-clover derivative, Dicoumarin, to prevent clotting in the repaired area, it is quite possible to reconnect arteries successfully. War surgeons, working under no such optimal conditions, tied off the artery with a strong ligature above and below the wound and removed the injured section, breaking the course of vasoconstrictor nerves traveling in the artery wall. Then they often did a strange thing. They tied off and cut the large vein beside the artery, whether it was involved in the injury or not.

Severing an uninjured vein doesn't make sense on superficial examination, but a consideration of the effect quickly makes it rational. A severed artery means less blood to the tissues and less oxygen. Blood contains much more oxygen than it normally gives to the tissue cells, however, largely because it stays in physico-chemical contact with cells for too short a period of time. Since there is less blood available, the next logical thing is to make it stay there longer. Severing the returning vein slows down the return flow, for now it, too, has to seek collateral channels, side roads by which to get back into the main channel. For the same reason the limb is not elevated on pillows; in severe cases it may even be kept dependent part of the time to encourage blood to remain in the limb for a longer period.

A few years ago, a lighted cradle would have been promptly placed over the injured extremity, with the explanation that heat dilated the blood vessels and increased blood flow. But heat does some other things that are not so good for a limb whose blood supply is low. It steps up metabolism, the rate at which a cell uses oxygen; it increases swelling and causes more pain; and it interferes with normal heat loss in the cell, which is having enough trouble getting rid of its waste products as it is. And so heat is no longer used. Papaverine, or similar drugs that cause vasodilation without ill effects, are injected regularly.

Along with all these things the vascular surgeon continues to block by novocain injection the sympathetic ganglia at intervals of every eight hours or so until the collateral channels have been well opened up and the limb is able to maintain its own circulation. Often, too, as soon as the operation is completed he packs the limb below the wound in ice. More about that later.

In many cases, injury to an artery may not sever the vessel but may so damage its wall that it later ruptures. The result is the same as if the artery were pierced. A large clot, or hematoma, tends to accumulate around the ruptured artery, increasing steadily in size until it shuts off the vessel by its own pressure. Pressure of the rhythmic thrusts of the blood column against this area may cause the hematoma to pulsate, giving the "pulsating hematoma" its name.

What usually happens is that the gradual wearing action of the blood escaping into the center of the hematoma hollows it out until, finally, a large sacular cavity is formed, filled with blood that swirls and eddies with each pulse beat. This is known as an aneurysm, although actually it differs from the true aneurysm following disease of the arterial wall.

The treatment of pulsating hematoma, or simple aneurysm, poses generally few problems for the vascular surgeon today. Many years ago Dr. Rudolph Matas, father of blood-vessel surgery, worked out the principles of treatment, emphasizing that the blood current into the weakened area must be shut off by tying and sectioning of the vessel above the aneurysm followed by removal of the entire sac if easily possible, or its obliteration by sewing the inside walls together. In some instances it is possible to reconstruct the inside of the sac to form a new channel, but this is not generally feasible. Aneurysms in general are allowed to go through a cooling-off period before operation; during this time the body generally develops its own by-pass or collateral circulation through side channels already present.

Before operating on an aneurysm the surgeon makes certain tests to determine whether it is safe to shut off the flow of blood through the sac and the vessel below it. Sometimes he applies pressure over the injured area to shut off the flow of blood for gradually longer periods, to encourage the development of collateral circulation. This is especially important when the aneurysm involves the great carotid channel to the head and brain.

Shutting off the flow of blood through the carotid artery for even a short period usually causes immediate fainting from anemia of the brain, but repeated periods of shutting off the blood flow accustom the brain to receiving its blood from the other side. When he can shut off the weakened channel completely without dangerously lowering the flow of blood to the extremity, the surgeon knows that he can operate safely. Under these circumstances there is rarely any ill effect from tying off the weakened artery and thus completely removing the danger, always present whenever there is an aneurysm, of sudden, fatal rupture. Removal of this constant threat of fatal hemorrhage is a result well worth taking great pains to accomplish.

Of far greater dramatic interest is a second type of aneurysm, which follows injury to both the artery and the vein. Since veins travel close beside the arteries almost everywhere in the body, these accidents are relatively frequent. Sometimes they result from rather insignificant injuries, such as a small stab wound with very little bleeding or a bullet wound that on superficial examination does not seem to involve any vital structure. War wounds produced many such aneurysms. Only in the weeks and months that follow does a set of symptoms and changes occur giving the characteristic picture of an arteriovenous aneurysm.

What actually takes place is that with openings in both artery and vein, blood under high pressure in the artery flows into the opening in the vein, where pressure is normally low. A pathway soon develops with a sac formed from a hematoma in much the same way that the sac forms when there is only rupture of an artery. This condition is called an arteriovenous aneurysm if a large sac is present, arteriovenous fistula if small. Depending on how far away the abnormal communication develops and the size of the vessel involved, the effect varies.

Always in these injuries the body seeks, by opening up collateral channels, to by-pass as much blood as possible and get it to the extremity where blood is badly needed, instead of going by a short cut through the abnormal opening into the venous system once more. In a small arteriovenous fistula in the finger of a child, the blood supply to that finger may be so enormously increased that it will grow much more rapidly and become markedly larger than its fellows. In a larger vessel supplying an extremity, the blood flow may be cut down to where the tissues are poorly nourished, and deep ulcerations or even gangrene may occur. Coupled with this the pressure from the arteries is interposed into the return of blood by way of the normal vein channels, exerting much the same effect as if the veins were obstructed and resulting in swelling, sometimes to a rather alarming degree. Nothing disturbs the circulation of an extremity quite so much as an arteriovenous communication.

But these local changes are by far the least important and dramatic links in the chain of symptoms that develop in the wake of one of these bizarre accidents. The by-passing of a large portion of the circulation by the escape of blood from the artery into the vein cuts down the total size of the entire circulatory system, while injecting into this diminished vein network a greater quantity of blood under pressure as it pours into the veins. The result is the equivalent of increasing to a great degree the amount of blood circulating through the entire system in any given period of time.

To take care of this increase in circulating blood volume the heart quickens its rate and steps up the blood pressure. A vicious cycle is set up, whereby blood is pumped faster toward the arteriovenous aneurysm, only to escape into the veins at a still faster rate, magnifying the whole change once more. Something has to give way if the vessels involved are large enough; usually it is the heart.

Unable to handle its greatly increased job, the heart begins to thicken, or hypertrophy. Gradually it enlarges, and as it does so its efficiency diminishes. A period is soon reached in which the heart begins to fail because of its inability to handle this constantly increasing output per minute. For this reason, more than because of its actual presence or its effect upon the limb involved, the abnormal by-pass must be removed, or the patient becomes a heart cripple.

The proof of this rather bizarre set of effects is simple. A hand laid over an arteriovenous aneurysm feels the purr of blood as it rushes through, a stethoscope placed on the skin over it hears the to-and-fro rush of blood with each pulse beat. But most dramatic of all is the result of simple pressure over the communication, shutting off the flow from artery to vein. Immediately the pulse slows, the blood pressure tends to become normal. This so-called "bradycardia effect" is a certain indication of an arteriovenous fistula or aneurysm.

Surgeons tackle this formidable operation when the larger vessels are concerned with a great deal of respect and preparation. First, the maximum collateral circulation must be developed. This usually means waiting for perhaps six months after the original injury before the operation is performed. Meanwhile the patient's general condition is improved to the highest possible degree, for the tissues around these areas are usually none too healthy from the prolonged disturbance in circulation and healing of operating wounds may be difficult. Also tests must be carried out to determine whether it is safe to shut off the flow through the artery, since such radical procedure is almost always necessary to cure this "Old Man of the Sea" riding and buffeting the circulation of the injured person. When it can be demonstrated by applying pressure over the artery that collateral circulation is satisfactory, the time to operate has arrived.

The neighborhood of an arteriovenous aneurysm is usually a maze of dilated blood vessels, the collateral network of the arteries and the vastly enlarged veins from the continual battering of arterial pressure into their normally placid currents. It is vital in these operations that the surgeon have complete control of this area of potential hemorrhage. To err once is to find the entire operative field flooded by a pool of blood.

These conditions frequently occur in areas that are extremely difficult to reach, such as behind the collar bone, or in the groin where the vessels of the leg dip deep into the body. The trained surgeon therefore first locates the artery both above and below the opening, and then the vein, also both above and below. With these secured he can set about closing the opening itself, an extremely difficult and rarely successful job, or he can remove the entire involved area, a much more certain way of achieving a cure.

Superficially it might seem simple to achieve a complete cure merely by stopping the flow of blood through the artery going to the abnormal communication, but this is an assumption that can only result in disaster. Shut off the artery above the arteriovenous aneurysm and blood immediately rushes through the collateral channels into the artery below the opening, from thence upward in the reverse direction and, still pursuing the path of least pressure, through the abnormal communication and into the vein. The effect is that of shutting off at once the entire blood supply to the extremity through the collateral channels, and gangrene will occur rapidly and practically always.

Half measures in treating these conditions will not be satisfactory; surgery is usually necessary. But the result is worth the time and the risk. With the blood from the arteries no longer leaking into the veins, the circulatory balance is restored. A boggy, painful, almost useless leg rapidly becomes normal, with blood once again flowing through its regular channels. The heart, deprived of its heavy burden, rapidly comes back to normal as a rule. The patient turns from a heart-conscious cripple back to a useful, healthy citizen.

Every day these miracles of blood-vessel surgery are being performed. During World War II the armed forces set up great centers in which trained specialists tackled these problems and daily transformed cripples into active men again. In these centers lessons were learned of tremendous value in the Atomic Age.

In a period when man is discovering newer and unbelievably effective weapons of destruction, it is encouraging to know that medical science is always entering new fields, where there are wide spaces yet to be conquered. There are, among others, the problems of heart circulation damaged by clotted coronary vessels, which we are only beginning to attack; heart valves, scarred and distorted by rheumatic fever and other disease, now just beginning to yield to the surgeon's scalpel; arteries shrunken and thickened by the dread Buerger's Disease, of which we know so little; blood vessels rupturing in the brain in the condition called apoplexy, with its sequelae of paralysis, coma, and death.

In two fields, branches of the new science of vascular surgery, great advances have been made. One is the use of cold in treating conditions that result in a lowered blood supply to body tissues; the other, less dramatic, but perhaps more important because the number of its victims is truly legion, is varicose veins.

12.

LIFE SUSPENDS AT ZERO

Crymotherapy, treatment by cold—Refrigeration anesthesia—Gangrene in diabetes and hardening of the arteries—Experiments with rats' tails—Effects of cold on tissues—Ice saves limbs—Trench foot—Other new uses of cold therapy—Can life be suspended by cold?

Medical history reveals that physicians of the ancient world appreciated the value of cold in relieving pain and reducing swelling. Interest in "crymotherapy," treatment of disease by means of cold, rose sharply in 1936 when Dr. Temple Fay, of Philadelphia, and his associates did some experimental work on the effect of lowered temperatures on persons suffering from inoperable cancer.

It had been previously observed that when cancers spread to other parts of the body by the seeding process called "metastasis," the new colonies usually grew in warmer areas. Other experimental work had suggested that cancer cells were more susceptible to damage by cold than normal body cells. Local application of ice to malignant growth had even resulted in a rather definite slowing in the rate of growth, as well as marked relief of pain.

The experiments of Fay and his group were widely reported in the newspapers. While not yielding anything that could be called a cure for cancer, their research did confirm previous observations of the effect of cold on body tissues. If they gave no new discovery to medical science, these experiments did serve as a stimulus for scientists to seek more knowledge in this hitherto little-studied field of crymotherapy.

127

And from them came the important technique of hypothermia, a method of lowering body temperatures during heart operations, which has given such spectacular results.

The benefit of refrigeration to tissues whose blood supply is diminished by disease or injury was something of an accidental discovery. For a long time it had been known that application of cold to living tissues for a short while paralyzed the pain nerve endings and thus achieved local anesthesia. A customary remedy for appendicitis has long been the application of ice caps to the abdomen, in the mistaken assumption that the appendix could be "frozen." Surgeons in general deplore this treatment, agreeing that cold does not penetrate deep enough to have much if any effect on the inflamed appendix. What it does do, however, is dull the nerve endings giving pain sensations, thus depriving the body of its main warning signal of impending disaster involving the appendix.

Chemicals that evaporate quickly, such as ether and ethyl chloride, are used to freeze the skin over boils and areas in which minor operations are to be performed. Cooling by ethyl-chloride spray is also of great value in treating acute sprains, bursitis, and similar conditions. In view of these effects, some surgeons began to reason that perhaps this idea of anesthesia by chilling could be applied on a larger scale, even to entire extremities, allowing operation without any other anesthetic.

Such an ambition was in no sense derived simply from a desire to experiment. Diabetes and arteriosclerosis, the hardening of the arteries associated with age, interfere greatly with the circulation of the toes, fingers, feet, and legs. Gangrene from insufficient blood supply is common in these cases. Many of the patients are among the very elderly and the poor, who usually do not present themselves for treatment until infections and malnutrition have weakened their resistance to an alarming degree. To save life, these infected or gangrenous limbs must often be removed quickly and mercifully. But in the weakened condition of these elderly sufferers from poor circulation, any anesthetic is dangerous, even spinal anesthesia, ordinarily quite safe for extremity work.

The ideal method of treatment in such cases would be to shut away from the rest of the body the infected limb and its gangrenous tissues until the general condition of the patient improved enough to allow amputation safely. But that means applying a tight tourniquet to the limb to shut off all blood flow, and the effect of tourniquets on extremities is well known. After a few hours, gangrene results, even in a normal limb.

Then a peculiar experiment gave an important clue. Strangely enough it dealt with rats' tails, and was reported in 1940 by Dr. B. Brooks and Dr. G. W. Duncan. They showed that the tails of rats, even when the entire blood supply was cut off by a tourniquet, could live for as long as ninety-six hours at 1° Centigrade, roughly freezing.

Exactly what happens when blood cells are exposed to cold is still not clear. One thing, however, seems definite. Cold slows down all the normal functions of living, until the cell seems to exist in a state of suspended animation. This suspension of life processes takes place apparently somewhere in the neighborhood of freezing. The important thing seems to be not how cold the tissue gets, but the rate at which it is brought back to normal temperature and the amount of oxygen available at this time.

Experience with trench foot, immersion foot, and frostbite has shown that freezing the tissue is not too important, so long as the return to normal temperature is not so rapid as to allow swelling and interfere with oxygenization of the cells during the recovery period.

Surgeons treating damaged tissues, however, do not try to lower the temperature of body cells to anything like freezing. The effects they wish to obtain occur at temperatures well above that level. Keeping in mind what was already known about the effect of cold on tissues damaged by poor blood supply and infection, it seemed safe to apply tourniquets to infected and gangrenous limbs and pack them in ice, or reduce the temperature by mechanical means, until the general condition of the patient improved to a point where amputation could be performed safely.

When this was done, the results amazed even the most sanguine observers. Not only was anesthesia complete in the superficial tissues, as would have been expected, but the entire limb could be severed with no more precautions than packing cotton into the patient's ears so he could not hear the saw cutting through bone. Amputations were performed with no after effects. The patients didn't even miss a meal, vitally important in keeping up the strength of their already poorly nourished bodies. Refrigeration anesthesia has been widely used for diabetes, arteriosclerosis, and similar degenerative diseases.

But anesthesia was not the only result of refrigeration. A number of other effects were noted. For one thing, pain disappeared almost completely soon after the application of ice, a result complete enough in itself for the pain was constant, boring, and often unbearable. Along with this local effect went a remarkable improvement in the patient's well-being, a lessening of the symptoms of toxic absorption accompanying the presence of an infected or gangrenous limb.

Sometimes removal of the stream of toxins pouring into the sick person's blood caused such a marked improvement that the operation could be safely postponed for several days to obtain maximum benefit. And, too, when the operation was performed, the surgeon often found that he could save much tissue that would ordinarily have been sacrificed.

With the improvement in general condition, the local situation grew better, too, and it was necessary only to remove minimal portions of gangrenous extremities. All this meant a new life for many diabetics, their limbs preserved for normal functions, once the diabetes was brought safely under control with the usual measures of diet and insulin.

From this observation of the effects of refrigeration on limbs to which a tourniquet had been applied, it was a natural step to test the effect on those without a tourniquet. Here the promise of earlier work was adequately fulfilled. When infected limbs, extremities in which the blood supply had been damaged by accidental injuries, were treated by refrigeration, the infection was often held in abeyance by the cold and absorption of toxins diminished. Interestingly enough, too, tissues that seemed lost from expected or beginning gangrene often came slowly back to normal.

Now, these tissues in infected and damaged limbs were not frozen; the temperatures were always well above the freezing point. The body cells were certainly not in the state of suspended animation that occurs at near freezing temperatures, so what brought about these beneficial effects?

While not yet completely understood, the facts seemed roughly as follows:

Application of cold decreases the metabolism of body cells, which means simply that the cell lives at a very much slower rate and therefore requires much less oxygen than at ordinary temperatures. In fact, at a level close to freezing, the oxygen consumption becomes almost zero. Whether in impending or actual gangrene from diabetes or arteriosclerosis, or from actual mechanical interruption of the blood flow to an extremity, the essential condition is lack of oxygen. Cutting down the need for oxygen makes supply and demand more nearly equal.

Ice also removes tissue heat by direct radiation at a time when the circulation is unable to remove it completely, and decreases the flow of fluid from the blood to the tissues, thus preventing swelling or decreasing it if already present. By cutting down blood flow and movement of tissue fluid, the absorption of poisons from infected and gangrenous tissues is markedly decreased. The relief of pain apparently occurs because of a direct effect of cold on the nerve endings themselves.

The obvious corollary to these observations was that whenever damage to a large artery interfered with the blood supply to an arm or a leg, packing the damaged extremity in ice should keep the oxygen needs at the lowest possible level until the circulation can be improved. This has proved to be true in many cases.

In the period between application of ice and surgery, the injury can be evaluated and the blood flow controlled if necessary by tourniquet. Then, sometimes through a new technique of replacing lost sections of the arteries with vitallium-metal tubes lined with vein sections, the flow of blood can be returned to the damaged limb. Meanwhile the effect of blood-vessel spasm, so often a deciding factor in arterial injuries, can be combated by injecting the deep nerve trunks beside the spine.

In one catastrophe that is a fairly frequent occurrence in some types of valvular heart disease, refrigeration has often proved lifesaving. In these cases, clots form inside the heart chambers, swirl through the valves, and are pumped out into the great arteries. Here they ride down the ever smaller branches until they strike a channel through which they cannot pass, usually in the arm or leg.

With circulation suddenly shut off by a blocked artery, the patient experiences agonizing pain, shock, and may lose the limb quite rapidly. Surgery can remove the clot if applied at once, but an operating room and blood-vessel surgeons are not always at hand. Since the surgeon is not immediately available, something is needed to preserve the limb until the patient can reach him. Packing in ice gives this protection in many cases, allowing the patient to be transported to a surgeon who can remove the clot. Limbs are often saved by this application of the life-suspending effects of cold on body tissues.

Paradoxically, in still another condition, trench foot, cold is both one of the main causative factors and a material aid in treatment.

The "Ardennes breakthrough" pinned many Allied troops into positions from which there was no immediate escape or relief, forcing them to remain often without food or changes of clothing for a week or more. Naturally, it brought a spate of trench foot, already a troublesome problem in the winter months in France before the breakthrough. The same thing happened in Korea, where conditions were equally rigorous. With the news of this unpleasant complication of modern warfare breaking on the radio and in the newspapers, trench foot might have been thought a new disease, but military doctors have known it intimately for more than a century.

Napoleon's surgeon, Baron Larrey, reported the effect of prolonged exposure to cold during the disastrous march on Moscow and described very accurately the condition we know as trench foot. The name derived from cases occurring in World War I, in which the conditions were peculiarly suitable for development of this painful affliction. Cold, we know now, is not the only factor. In fact, it is only one of several. Cases have been reported of so-called "immersion foot" occurring in shipwrecked men in southern waters.

Immersion foot is now recognized to be similar, if not identical, with trench foot. Dependent position, constricting clothing, and other factors are apparently as important as cold, probably even more so, in causing these unhappy complications of warfare.

Eskimo folklore and the experience of Arctic explorers and others exposed to cold for prolonged periods, all bear out the concept of trench foot as an affliction not limited in any sense to warfare. Mechanized battle conditions did not tend to produce trench foot to any great degree; it was only when conditions became static in cold weather that the injury came suddenly to the forefront.

Symptoms of trench foot may appear anywhere, even in interior zones, whenever conditions favor its occurrence. It has been produced experimentally in rabbits by prolonged exposure to damp cold. Frostbite, differing from trench foot only in that there is actual freezing rather than simple cooling of tissues, happens frequently to workers employed by the City of New York in winter.

Lowered temperatures are far from being the only factor in causing trench foot. Tissue cultures, cells growing in test tubes, have been subjected to temperatures down to freezing without affecting their growth in any perceptible way. Many investigators believe that permanent damage to living tissue occurs when their temperature is reduced as low as 23° Fahrenheit. On the other hand, human spermatozoa, ordinarily very susceptible to injury, have been subjected to temperatures as low as a hundred and more degrees below zero and subsequently thawed and found perfectly viable. Fish survive after being frozen in solid ice, provided they are slowly thawed.

Newspapers reported in 1020 the finding of a prehistoric mammal frozen in the earth in Siberia for thousands of years, the meat being perfectly preserved and suitable for feeding to the dogs. Living bacteria were cultured from the trunk of the mammoth, evidence that life can be preserved for thousands of years in the frozen state. It is not simply cold, then, that produces such painful afflictions as trench foot. Scientists generally agree now as to the mechanism by which trench foot and immersion foot occur. Experiments show that subjection to temperatures below 50° Fahrenheit for more than twelve hours will damage tissue when certain other conditions are present. These conditions, all occurring in fixed types of warfare under unsatisfactory situations, are (1) obstruction to the circulation; (2) slight pressure, particularly if unevenly applied; and (3) subsequent warming. These factors deserve a few words of explanation.

Obstruction to the circulation does not necessarily mean an unsatisfactory shoe, and the fact that the toes are the parts most affected means nothing, for the circulation in the toes is generally inferior to that in the rest of the extremity. Garters will give the same obstructive effect, and in shipwreck survivors, often barefoot, the only obstruction to the circulation was possibly by the pressure of the lifeboat seats against the relatively exposed arteries in the popliteal space back of the knee.

Most writers agree that dependency alone is the most pertinent factor as far as obstruction to the circulation goes in producing trench foot. Prolonged immobility of the leg in the dependent position will markedly decrease blood flow; this is probably the main reason for circulatory interference in men forced to lie or stand in trenches, foxholes, or behind barricades. Dependency is perhaps the most important factor —even more important than cold—in the occurrence of immersion foot in shipwrecked or torpedoed sailors in southern waters. Here the cooling seems to be by evaporation from the skin, particularly at night, when the physical process of evaporation known as "supercooling" may lower skin temperature well below the 50° Fahrenheit level believed by many investigators to be the critical point for development of trench foot.

The effect of pressure on any damaged tissue is well known, as witness the development of bed sores in paralysis cases and others in which the tissues have been damaged. Classical example of this is the varicose ulcer, an accompaniment of the poor circulation resulting from the pooling of blood in dilated varicose veins.

Undoubtedly most important of all in the development of trench foot is subsequent warming of the extremity after long exposure to "wet cold." It must be emphasized again that it is wet cold that does the most damage. Just why wet cold should be more damaging than dry is not immediately apparent, but investigators agree that water on the skin acts as a conducting agent for the cold in addition to its part in the normal cooling effect of evaporation. Between the two, a much lower temperature is obtained than with dry cold alone. In either event, subsequent warming sets up a train of events that may well result in irreparable damage to the already injured tissues.

Gradual thawing of frozen or damaged tissues has long been recognized as essential to recovery. Eskimos know this, and the lore of the Gloucester fishermen, working under unbelievably terrible conditions of wet and cold while fishing off the Grand Banks, includes treating frostbite by application of cold. This treating of cold with cold, like fighting fire with fire, is completely reasonable when considered in the light of our modern scientific knowledge of crymotherapy.

Most patients do not reach a doctor until they have already removed their shoes and allowed their feet to become warm. Thus they have started the chain of events that may result in disaster. There can be no doubt that warming an overcool foot damages it far more than the original cooling, by causing swelling which interferes with the circulation and proper nutrition of the already damaged cells.

Eskimos recognized this a long time ago when they handed down the legend of treating frozen feet with snow. Under suitable conditions war surgeons like to treat trench foot by cooling, allowing the temperature to rise slowly, giving the tissues time to adjust themselves slowly as the temperature returns to normal.

A certain number of cases have been treated by refrigeration and a very gradual raising of the temperature to normal. One method is by exposing the feet to dry, cool air flowing over them, raising the temperature very gradually over a period of days to the normal level. Cases treated in this way have shown markedly less tissue damage than those warmed quickly to normal temperatures.

Great though the advances in our knowledge have been in the past ten years, the field of refrigeration therapy with various degrees of cold has probably only been touched. It is now known that heat is not indicated in the treatment of traumatic shock in every case, that instead a certain amount of cold, properly controlled, may preserve the blood-vessel spasm, which is a protecting measure in severe shock. In burns, too, cold has proved effective in relieving pain, preventing swelling, and promoting healing.

Certainly in the future new frontiers in surgery will be opened by our knowledge of crymotherapy, just as a new frontier in heart surgery has apparently been opened by the use of low temperatures to preserve brain cells during periods in which it is necessary to shut away the flow of blood while the heart is being repaired.

Who knows? Some day it may be possible to suspend life at zero for entire human bodies.

13.

VARICOSE VEINS

*Wide incidence of varicose veins, with ulcers,
and eczema—How they develop—Heredity—
Treatment by injections—Dangers of phlebitis—
The operation for varicose veins*

Probably no disease affects so large a portion of the
population and yet, as commonly treated, yields such uniformly poor results as varicose veins of the leg and their more
serious sequels, varicose ulcer and varicose eczema, both degrees of the same process. The reason for this can be traced
generally to incomplete methods of treatment, conditioned
largely by the failure of both patient and doctor to appre-
ciate the fundamentally simple considerations that govern
the formation and development of these diseased and weakened blood vessels. Yet no condition is simpler to explain,
simpler to treat, once the problem is approached, as should
be all surgical problems, with full appreciation of first, the
anatomy of the veins of the lower extremity, and second,
the hydrostatic-pressure peculiarities that they, more than the
rest of the venous system, exhibit. Rightly treated, varicose
veins, even with ulcer, can be completely cleared up in a matter of weeks by a combination of surgical skill and the products of modern scientific research.

To understand how varicose veins are attacked by modern surgical scientists, let us first see how they are formed.
The veins of the body form one half of the orderly maze of
circulatory channels through which the blood flows. The arteries form the other half. In the arteries the blood pressure
is high, a force imparted to the moving stream by the mus-

cular pump, the heart, that stands at the center of the circulatory system. As the heart forces blood into the arteries, the walls, which contain elastic tissue, are distended by the pulsing flow of blood. It is this rhythmic distension of the arteries that is distinguishable as the pulse at the wrist and the temple, as well as in other less easily felt vessels. The elastic recoil of the artery walls on the blood they contain adds its force to the pressure given the moving stream of blood by the heart. These two forces together, combined with the resistance of smaller and smaller arteries as the blood progresses away from the heart, sustain the blood pressure in the arterial system.

When blood reaches the veins, however, the pressure of the arteries has been largely expended and blood must then find its way back to the heart by other means. Consider that man, in the process of evolution, has become an erect instead of a four-footed animal and you can easily see what a problem in hydrodynamics it becomes to lift the blood some three and a half to four feet to the level of the heart. Obviously, some special considerations must enter into the function of the circulation, if the blood is not to stagnate in the veins.

Ingeniously enough, the body seeks to overcome this difficulty of lifting a blood column to the heart by placing the main blood channels deep within the muscular portions of the extremities. Here they are continually subject to the massaging action of muscles in motion, shoving the blood up the long, thin-walled veins toward the heart. At regular intervals along the veins of the legs, ingenious valves, infoldings of the lining membrane of the blood vessel, let the blood through on the way to the heart, but close against it when it seeks to flow backward toward the toes. So long as these valves continue to function correctly, blood cannot leak back and its movement toward the heart is expedited.

In addition to the deep vein channels, however, there is another network of veins in the legs which lies just beneath the skin. These are normally easily seen over the surface of the foot, or in individuals with pale skins the entire network can be visualized as a bluish pattern of vessels through the skin itself.

The superficial veins remove blood from the skin and ex-

ternal tissues. Gradually as they approach the knee, the channels join into two larger veins that empty into the deep vessels at the groin. The manner of emptying here varies greatly,
and unless the surgeon is familiar with these variations, he
may fail at the very beginning in his attempt to cure the
patient.

Sometimes only one vein, called the internal or great saphenous, brings blood from the entire superficial network of the
veins and delivers it into the deep channels at the groin.
More often, two or more larger channels carry the flow. Between the superficial and the deep vein channels there also
exists a number of connecting veins, ordinarily called "communicating vessels." These communicating veins—there are
usually three or four below the knee and almost always at
least two above it—carry off part of the blood from the superficial network and, perforating the muscles, enter the deep
vessels far beneath. In these communicating veins, too, there
are valves to prevent a back flow and thus promote the emptying of blood from the superficial vessels, which do not have
muscle massaging to aid in their work.

Keeping in mind the relationship of these two networks,
the superficial and the deep, and the communicating vessels
between them, and bearing in mind the importance of the
valves in keeping the blood flowing through them in the right
direction, it is quite simple to understand how varicose veins
occur and, understanding this, to plan a logical and effective
method of treatment.

Anatomy and physiology have repeatedly demonstrated the
basic scientific truth that man was never meant to stand erect;
the placing of many of his organs shows this. But since he has
assumed the erect posture, the dynamics of his circulation
have been correspondingly altered. Placing the deep veins
where they will be massaged by muscular action removes
blood from the lower extremities. To carry it through the
trunk to the heart, other factors must now come into play. The
most important of these are changes in pressure that occur
with respiration.

The trunk is composed essentially of a compartment divided into two sections, the chest and abdomen. Between
them is a movable partition, the diaphragm. When air is

taken into the lungs, the chest expands in its front-to-back diameter by moving the ribs upward and outward, while at the same time it expands in its vertical length by moving the diaphragm downward. This creates a vacuum, or negative pressure, in the chest, which causes air to be sucked into the lungs. At the same time this negative pressure causes blood to be drawn up through the great veins of the trunk and into the heart. But this is not the entire effect of respiration, for when the diaphragm moves downward, it decreases the size of the abdominal cavity and thus raises the pressure inside the abdomen. This increased abdominal pressure is transmitted through the thin walls of the veins and also forces blood upward into the chest.

Thus respiration pulls blood into the chest by negative pressure and pushes it out of the abdomen by positive pressure. Since the valves in the leg veins keep blood from being forced downward into the limbs, it has to go upward toward the heart; there isn't anywhere else for it to go. Were all this not true, blood would flow backward and stagnate in the veins of the legs.

This is exactly what tends to happen in people who work long hours standing in one place with relatively little muscular activity of the legs. Very much the same thing happens to the lower legs when one sits for long hours with the feet hanging down. An additional factor is the pressure of a chair, or a foot rest on a hospital bed, against the veins in the exposed position in the popliteal space back of the knee. When the veins remain filled with turgid blood for a long time, their walls tend to stretch and dilate. As they do, they set up a mild inflammation in their walls.

Gradually, then, the veins become large and tortuous, lifting up the skin in a manner resembling the path of a mole through the garden. This is the typical appearance of varicose veins.

But the damage does not stop at merely dilating the veins. As the vessels continue to expand, the valves, too, become stretched and soon reach a point where they are no longer able to hold up the column of blood above them. Blood then leaks backward, and the veins just below the varicosed area are subjected to increased pressure, and soon join those above in exhibiting the dilated, tortuous pattern characteristic of varicose veins. Thus it is easy to see that once varicosities start developing, they tend to progress, until the entire superficial circulation of the leg is involved.

Position is not the only cause of varicose veins, however. Heredity undoubtedly plays a part. Pregnancy, when the enlarging uterus presses on the pelvic veins and interferes with their emptying, is also a potent cause of varicose veins. Every obstetrician is familiar with the fact that his patients during pregnancy often show dilated veins, which disappear when the child is born. Many obstetricians insist that patients with a tendency toward varicose veins wear elastic stockings during pregnancy. The stocking, briefly, presses on the superficial veins to prevent them from dilating and forces the blood, which would ordinarily accumulate in the superficial network, through the communicating veins into the deeper channels.

As varicose veins begin to form, however, still another factor comes into play. A most important factor it is, too, for unless it is taken into consideration, treatment will be a failure. Blood-vessel surgeons feel that the failure to recognize changes that have taken place in the valves of the communicating veins is responsible for a large part of the failures to cure, which have given the treatment of varicose veins a bad name.

As the varicose veins begin to dilate, the valves between these two great systems of blood vessels in the legs also tend to break down. Now blood flows into the deep vessels but, since the valves are not working properly, surges right back into the dilated superficial system. Blood-vessel surgeons call these areas "blowouts." Unless they are treated, ordinary methods of curing varicose veins by injection, or by operation plus injecting, will fail completely. More about that later.

But does this explanation, covering the development of the dilated veins, also explain the ulcers that so often accompany varicose veins, frequently resisting treatment for years? Quite simply, it does.

Blood going to tissues through the arteries carries food and oxygen; blood leaving the tissues by way of the veins carries waste products, including carbon dioxide. It is quite as important to remove the waste as to provide food and oxygen. Without the latter, the cell dies; with too much of the former, the same thing occurs. Thus when blood is not properly removed from the tissues by the veins, it stagnates. Swelling then occurs, there is lack of a fresh supply of oxygen, and an accumulation of waste products. This is exactly what happens in severe varicose veins. Over a long period, the tissues, particularly the skin of the feet and the ankles, become less and less healthy. Eruptions may occur, and skin inflammations are followed by great weeping, irritated, discolored areas, which are called varicose eczema.

More often, however, the skin may be bruised by an injury ordinarily as innocuous as striking a shin against a chair in the dark. The wounded area then breaks down, fails to heal, and a chronic ulcer forms. Quite often the unhappy sufferer, not realizing the basic cause, tries to treat the ulcer without treating the condition that caused it. Salves and unguents, advertised by legions in the newspapers every day, are applied, often damaging the unhealthy tissues even further with the chemicals they contain. The limping patient rapidly becomes discouraged—especially if some physician, with honest if misguided enthusiasm, gives him a series of injections with the assurance that a cure will be forthcoming immediately, and fails.

The reason for the failure to cure is obvious by now even to the casual reader. The ulcer cannot be cured until the underlying stagnation of blood in the tissues, with its accompanying features of oxygen-lack and waste accumulation, are removed. Remove them and the ulcer will cure itself in almost every case.

How, then, should varicose veins be treated?

There is nothing complicated about the method successfully used in blood-vessel clinics all over the country. It consists essentially of two procedures, in most cases carried out simultaneously. The first is to interrupt surgically the back flow of blood from the deep veins of the legs into the dilated, tortuous varicose vessels of the superficial vein network. The second is to inject into the empty, diseased veins a mildly irritating chemical that causes the blood-vessel walls to adhere tightly together, obliterating the dilated superficial channels and forcing blood into the deeper normal veins where the muscular action, coupled with the pressure changes in the trunk, will insure the movement of blood back to the heart. In simple cases, where the section of vein involved is small, injections alone may be all that is necessary, but blood-vessel surgeons are coming to believe more and more that this is rarely the case.

Before recommending and performing the very simple, even minor, operations that cure varicose veins, the surgeon must know several things about the patient. First he must be certain that the deep veins are open. Phlebitis, that dangerous and occasionally fatal deep-vein inflammation, which sometimes follows pregnancy or operations, may result in blood clots closing off the deep vessels. The resulting dilation of the superficial veins to carry the complete blood load gives them the appearance of varicose veins, but to treat them on that basis may be disastrous. So the blood-vessel surgeon performs a few simple tests to discover whether the deep vessels are performing normally. Quite simply this can be done by applying a snug elastic bandage to the entire leg and letting the patient walk around for about an hour. If the deep veins are not open, pain, cramping, and acute discomfort will identify the condition within a few minutes, since the return of blood to the heart is largely shut off from that extremity by collapsing the superficial veins.

A second test tells the surgeon how extensive his operation will have to be. Formerly several tests were used, but they were sometimes confusing. More recently an all-purpose examination, called the "multiple tourniquet test," has been devised to give the surgeon all the information he needs.

In the multiple tourniquet test, the patient stands until the diseased veins are filled with blood. A soft rubber or elastic tourniquet is then placed around the upper thigh and drawn tight enough to block the dilated veins, but not to obstruct the flow through the artery. Relatively light pressure is necessary; if the patient complains of numbness from the tourniquet, it is too tight. Then the patient exercises for about a minute, doing deep knee bends, with the tourniquet in place all the while. With muscular action, the dilated superficial veins will empty themselves through the communicating vessels and the varicose veins will collapse as the blood leaves them.

When the patient stops exercising, the easily visible veins should fill quite slowly in about a minute, if the valves in the communicating veins are functioning correctly. If they are not, there will be a visible back flow of blood into the varicose veins at the level where the valves of the communicating vessels are poor. Locating this back flow is the most important feature of the test, for if there is a blowout that is not recognized and taken care of in the subsequent operation, treatment will practically always fail.

Sometimes, in severe cases, there are several of these blowouts. This is liable particularly to be true in cases in which ulcers have developed. Each blowout must be located by applying the tourniquet at successively lower levels and watching the filling of the varicose veins after exercise. One method of performing the test puts three or four tourniquets on at one time to locate the blowouts more rapidly. Whatever the method used, each communicating vein in which the valves are not functioning must be located at its connection with the superficial veins and carefully marked for direct attack at the time of operation.

Knowing the exact status of the situation now, the surgeon is ready to operate. He makes a small incision in the crease of the groin, high up. Usually the operation is carried out under local anesthesia, since most surgeons prefer their patients to start walking immediately after the operation. The great saphenous vein, which drains most of the superficial network, is tied off and cut where it enters the deep channels at the groin. All other branches entering here, usually three to five in number, are also tied off and cut. The incision is small, the scar not even noticeable when placed in the fold of the skin, as it usually is.

Sometimes the chemical solution used to obliterate the varicose veins is injected downward into them at this point. Many surgeons, however, prefer to make a second small incision over the saphenous vein at the inner side of the knee, pick it up, tie and cut it here, and inject downward into the lower leg. If this is done, a pressure bandage is applied immediately after the injection to bring the irritated vein walls into contact and prevent them from becoming filled by painful clots from the irritant action of the injection solution. The patient then walks, thereby squeezing excess solution into the deep veins, where it is taken away by the moving blood current and harmlessly diluted in the blood stream.

Not to let the patient walk immediately may prove dangerous—another reason why the operation is performed under local anesthesia—for if the irritating solution puddles in the deep veins, they, too, may be damaged, a distinctly undesirable complication.

Many blood-vessel surgeons prefer not to perform injections at the time of operation, but carry out whatever subsequent injections are necessary at a later date.

Most important of all, if blowouts are present, small incisions must be made over them and they must be tied off and cut as they perforate the muscles on the way to the deep veins. If properly located and marked off beforehand, this can be accomplished rapidly. In unusually severe cases, surgeons have recently begun to strip the dilated, tortuous veins from beneath the skin, removing them entirely through many small incisions.

In the case of varicose ulcer, treatments must necessarily be more prolonged. One frequent cause of ulcer is a blowout close to the ulcer that goes unrecognized because the skin near varicose ulcers often becomes so thick that the vein cannot be seen. An ingenious method of demonstrating such a vessel has been devised. It consists of injecting into the superficial veins of the lower leg a solution of Diodrast, or some similar chemical, which casts a shadow on the X-ray and is used in photographing the interior of the kidney pelvis. Injected into the veins of the leg, Diodrast gives an X-ray picture of the entire venous network of the leg, a great help in severe ulcer cases.

Ulcer patients are usually treated before the operation by pressure bandages; often a white boot called an "Unna Paste" boot is used. More recently, elastic and even plastic bandages are used. The purpose is to collapse the varicose veins and improve the circulation of the tissues around the ulcer before treating the underlying varicose veins, which caused it.

Often a pressure boot and taking the patient off her feet for a few weeks improves the circulation so quickly that the ulcer heals spontaneously. To be led into the mistaken belief that no other treatment is necessary only means a recurrence. Healing the ulcer by compression and rest is a temporary stopgap only; a cure can be accomplished only by carrying the treatment to its completion, particularly by operation and by carefully severing all blowouts at the same time.

It is not certain just how much can be done to prevent varicose veins. Wearing elastic stockings during pregnancy almost certainly does help. Accumulation of excess fat is certainly a handicap; many severe cases occur in very fat women.

Persons who work at jobs that require long standing in one position should go out of their way to move around frequently, do a few knee bends or otherwise stimulate the muscles that massage blood through the deep veins. Tight garters undoubtedly further the development of varicosities and should not be worn by women who tend to develop varicose veins or whose families exhibit any definite hereditary tendency toward them. Once the veins begin to develop, elastic stockings will do much to take the strain off weak vein walls. Many persons with severe varicose veins find that they need no other treatment.

One very present danger to persons with dilated veins is rupture of a blood-filled vessel by a blow, or small cut, or sometimes spontaneously. Many persons have bled to death, quite needlessly, from such an accident. Pressure with the hand, a handkerchief, a towel, applied tightly enough directly over the bleeding area will stop the flow of blood. Pressure with the fingers above and below the bleeding area will stop the flow at once. Failing these, the prone position with the feet elevated vertically will also stop the blood loss at once, until a pressure dressing can be applied. There should be no excuse for severe hemorrhage from varicose veins.

Once the varicosities develop and start causing serious symptoms, the simplest and quickest way to complete recovery is usually through ligation and injection. Injection alone will cure mild cases, but one must be certain of the condition. When in doubt, combining a small operation (one frequently performed in the outpatient clinic) with the injection is certain to cure. There is no excuse for the pessimism with which varicose veins are generally regarded. The application of simple principles of blood-vessel surgery will insure a cure in practically every case.

But there is still another way in which the new knowledge of vascular surgery insures the patient, and that is by protecting against the complications that may follow any operation . . . by making operations safe.

14.

MAKING OPERATIONS SAFE

*Safety of surgery today—Remaining dangers—
Pulmonary embolus—Treatment—X-rays and
venography*

No operation is entirely without danger; every surgeon learns that fact early in his career and acquires a healthy respect for the many factors that may influence the outcome of even the simplest procedure. Less than a century ago the hospitals of Europe, the famed Hotel Dieu of Paris, the Allgemeines Krankenhaus of Vienna, and similar institutions throughout the world were in many respects charnel houses from which many patients never returned. Through them stalked the twin specters of infection and inflammation; in their wake was the grim figure of death. So prevalent was infection that statistics recently gathered by an obstetrical writer show indubitably that it was safer for a woman to be gored by a bull and thus delivered of her child than to submit to a Caesarean operation in what were then the leading lying-in hospitals of Europe.

The last twenty years have seen surgery become safer and safer, the mortality rate from strictly operative cases brought lower and lower, as each barrier has been surmounted. But one cause of death following operations long baffled the doctors. It was a dramatic sort of death, occurring usually just as the patient began to get out of the bed, or even on the morning of discharge from the hospital. One minute he was laughing, talking, the next there was a gasp, a fighting for breath, a sudden telltale blueness of lips and ear lobes, a sharp breath-stopping pain—and death, sudden and inexplicable to the family, who had thought all danger past.

This death was easily explainable at the autopsy table, however; the cause was there for all to see—a dark red blood clot, filling the vessels to one section of the lung and shutting off the function of oxygen transmission as effectively as if a valve had been turned in the oxygen-supply mechanism—as indeed it had. Even so, this embolus—the medical name for any foreign substance traveling in the blood stream to cause obstruction to arteries, whose diameters are too small to allow it to pass through—usually did not involve both lungs.

Why, then, could not the other lung satisfy the oxygen needs of the body? People lived with one lung collapsed because of tuberculosis, with one lung removed because of cancer. The answer is not yet completely known. Probably it lies in a peculiar sort of reaction set up in a blood vessel that survives an insult, whether a wound, an irritating chemical, or sudden blockage by a blood clot.

This reaction of blood-vessel spasm has been seen by war surgeons in battle wounds involving blood vessels or in their immediate proximity. The intense spasm of blood vessels not only at the point of injury but over a wide area has already been described in connection with vascular wounds. Why is it not reasonable to deduce that the shock of a blood clot traveling in the blood stream and lodging in an artery causes a widespread spasm of other arteries of the lungs, shutting down momentarily the entire function of those organs without whose proper action life ceases in a matter of minutes? It is a logical explanation, well within our present knowledge of what happens in blood-vessel obstruction in other areas.

Embolus blocking of the leg arteries, a fairly frequent concomitant of some forms of heart disease, results in a widespread spasm, blocking the blood oxygen supply to an arm or leg. Relief of the spasm by injection of the sympathetic nerves that control the blood vessels materially lowers the necessity for amputation in these cases, even allows surgical opening of the obstructed artery and removal of the clot.

Why, then, cannot the lung arteries be protected from spasm, too, by injection of the sympathetic nerves deep in the neck and upper chest? Perhaps they can, when more is known about exactly what happens; perhaps many cases may even be saved in this way. But pulmonary, or lung, embolism is usually so rapidly fatal that there is not time to make injections; in most cases there is hardly time to call the doctor. That method seems out—for the time being, anyway.

For years doctors sought to attack the embolus problem in yet another way, by immediate operation and removal of the clot from the arteries going to the lungs. A famous pioneer surgeon many years ago originated an operation that he was able to perform, but only in rare instances successfully. Others have tried and almost uniformly failed, with the result that the operation has been practically given up in recent years. It is a heroic sort of operation: a quick incision in the chest over the great blood vessels just above the heart, a tourniquet around the arteries to the lungs just where they leave the heart, an incision into the artery, and extraction of the blood clot. For success it requires an operating force constantly ready, a surgeon of rare skill, a mobilizing of forces on a split-second schedule practically impossible to obtain. It is not surprising, then, that few of these operations have been attempted, almost none successfully.

But surgeons did not accept the dictum that pulmonary embolism was impossible to prevent. They began to search for causes, ways to tell when a patient was going to develop a blood clot, methods of stopping it before it ever reached the lungs, the danger spot. In the great clinics of the country, research specialists studied the circulation after operations, kept records of the occurrence of fatal and nonfatal lung clots. Many things were tried to prevent their occurrence, too, for it was recognized that the whole problem was tied up somehow with another great postoperative enigma. This is the strange inflammation of the leg veins that sometimes follows childbirth and, less often, surgical operation.

Surgeons were familiar with this picture of phlebitis, or, as it is correctly called, "femoral thrombophlebitis"—inflammation of the leg veins with clot formation. It, too, happened with no apparent cause. A patient would be progressing normally after an operation or delivery; then one night there was a pain, not always severe, in the calf or thigh. The following morning the leg was swollen, red, tender. The patient's temperature went up and the by-products of fever and inflammation, headache, loss of appetite, drowsiness, appeared. Occasionally, too, if a nurse happened to make a mistake in these cases of mild leg pain and rubbed the thigh, a blood clot was apparently milked out of the great leg veins and into the circulation, where it traveled in the blood stream and through it to the lungs as an embolus.

So in every hospital the dictum was set up: never rub the legs of postoperative patients who complained of leg pain.

If this phlebitis problem had been as simple as that, there wouldn't have been much to it. A few days of swelling and fever, a little pain, then a subsidence of the whole condition. But it wasn't; for it sometimes went on for weeks and subsided only gradually then. Often one leg was left permanently larger than the other, the circulation in the veins and lymphatic vessels was permanently damaged so that the leg became boggy, swollen, ungainly, often marred by unsightly discolorations and ulcers and by widely dilated superficial veins. Patients didn't like this complication and usually blamed the surgeon.

So surgeons sought to prevent phlebitis and in so doing soon recognized that they were attacking the embolus problem. If the clots in legs infected by phlebitis sometimes broke off and became lung emboli, then it was logical to say that pulmonary embolus came from phlebitis. The trouble was that in only a very few cases of death from embolus was there an actual demonstrable phlebitis of the legs, characterized by the known signs of pain, swelling, redness, and general malaise.

But the study of the leg-vein inflammation was not entirely fruitless. As they began to pay more attention to what went on in these inflamed veins, doctors began to get a little better idea of what happened. They began to see the cases earlier and they saw now a picture, often only a few hours in duration, that they hadn't seen before.

These cases at the first sign of leg pain did not yet show swelling and redness; more commonly they looked pale, as if something had shut off the flow through the arteries, which were not directly affected by the inflammation of the veins. In fact, they looked very much as if an embolus had blocked an artery instead of a vein; only later did the signs of vein obstruction appear.

Doctors were not completely conscious of the role of the sympathetic nervous system in controlling the flow of blood through arteries and veins, until comparatively recent times. And so it was only a few years ago that the real sequence of events in these painful cases of phlebitis became clear. It was simple then to explain: in some way the vein became inflamed, setting up a widespread spasm of the blood vessels, obstructing the proper return of blood to the vein side of the circulation, resulting in swelling, pain, and other signs usually associated with a true thrombophlebitis.

Knowing this, they had a plan of attack now. Inject the sympathetic nerves—easily accessible as small accumulations of nerve tissue in the lower back called ganglia—and stop this spasm of the blood vessels; that should at least remove the symptoms of phlebitis. This in itself would be something, for the condition is often very painful, and always a shock to the morale of a patient recovering from a serious operation.

Many surgeons began treating these cases of leg-vein inflammation with novocain injections to the lower back, blocking out the nerves that controlled the blood vessels of the affected limb. It was an experiment, but like all medical experiments on human beings, done only after the results were practically certain. And the results exceeded even the fondest hopes of the investigators.

In the usual picture of phlebitis, a patient develops a painful, tender, red swollen leg perhaps in the middle of the night. The temperature shoots up, all the unpleasant by-products of inflammation appear in the form of pain, headache, and feeling-bad-all-over. Everything, according to previous experience, points to many weeks of sickness, perhaps a leg permanently crippled—particularly undesirable in a woman, and many of these patients are women.

Now the surgeon takes four slender, flexible needles and a syringe and novocain. He turns the patient on the side or face, locates the tips of the spine that project from the vertebrae in the lower back, and measures a space the breadth of two fingers away from each. Here he makes a tiny wheal of novocain on the side of the affected leg, and inserts a needle painlessly, probing deep into the tissues until the needle strikes against the bodies of the vertebrae. Into each of the four needles he injects novocain, then removes them.

With the needles out, the patient is turned and the limb is studied. Soon there is a definite flushing, as constricted blood vessels open up to allow free flow of blood; the limb takes on a perceptible warmth and pain disappears almost like magic. That in itself is an end, but here it is only the beginning. Every twelve, or perhaps eight, hours, the injections are repeated; the patient may even be allowed to walk with the help of an elastic bandage. Temperature falls, the inflammation disappears, swelling melts away. In most cases the entire disturbance seems to disappear in a matter almost of days, certainly fewer days than the weeks and months during which many cases were crippled before this simple new treatment was discovered.

The problem of acute thrombophlebitis was conquered by this simple method. Even the chronic form has been benefited, often cured by these same injections. Patients whose legs have been swollen for months sometimes find the size returning to normal after only a few injections.

But what did all this have to do with the problem of death from embolism in the lungs?

The answer lay, paradoxically enough, in the discovery that this form of blood-vessel inflammation, in which clots blocked the veins, rarely did cause embolus formation. There was something about these clots associated with inflammation that seemed to seal them to the walls of the vessels—perhaps it was the very inflammatory process. But there was another group with less severe symptoms and with little if any inflammation of the veins, cases to which little attention would have been called or that perhaps would have been overlooked entirely except for one thing—these were the ones that developed emboli. These mild vein cases were the ones associated with sudden death.

When surgeons grasped that essential truth, the problem of embolus formation was practically licked. It required only the same application of the principles learned in treating blood-vessel disturbances elsewhere, the same kind of thinking that had led to the use of sympathetic injections in the thrombophlebitis cases, to develop methods of breaking down this last great barrier to making operations really safe.

While doctors were correlating these facts about leg-vein inflammation, they were also studying the embolus cases themselves. They quickly saw that not everyone who had a disturbance of the leg-vein circulation developed an embolus, but they also found that many who did not have any demonstrable leg-vein involvement did have emboli. How, then, could they go about predicting who would get in trouble and who wouldn't?

Statistics in medicine are often misleading, especially if they don't cover enough territory. That's why a competent researcher studies not only his own results but also the published results of others who have been working on the same problem. From a broad study like this, investigators at Tulane, Harvard, Johns Hopkins, and other famous schools arrived at some valuable conclusions. The most important was that about 70 per cent of all fatal cases of lung embolus occur in patients past fifty years of age. That was important because doctors could make a closer search in these patients. But another conclusion was even more important.

Seventy per cent of those who die have a warning embolus before!

These were important figures, startling figures. They meant that embolus was not the stalker-by-night, the striker-in-the-darkness-without-warning, that it was generally conceived to be. To a certain degree, the likelihood of its occurrence could be predicted. These warning emboli were not always the dramatic, shocking occurrences like the ones that caused death. More often they were attacks that less observant doctors might label "pleurisy" or a "slight pneumonia."

Even in the X-ray these little accidents didn't immediately show up; often there would be merely a faint shadow that only the expert student of lung X-rays would recognize as abnormal. But to the trained surgeon, always carrying in his mind the possibilities of what might happen, the warning emboli could be recognized for what they were, small clots traveling in the blood stream and blocking off a section of the lung, usually a wedge-shaped area at the bottom of the lung. Having satisfied himself that an embolus had actually occurred, the surgeon could then make an important conclusion:

There was about a three-to-one chance that another embolus would occur, this time more probably fatal.

But it wouldn't be much comfort to the patient to know what his chances of catastrophe were. What was needed was a method of protecting those three out of four patients from that second, often fatal embolus. And there's where the whole problem of lung clot and leg-vein clot tied in, for they were simply effect and cause, in the order named.

Surgeons everywhere began to study these cases of warning embolus; better than that, they began to watch all their cases, especially those in the upper age groups, for a sign of clot formation in the leg veins. And they found that usually when a patient had chest pain and fever a few days after operation, with the signs of a small pulmonary embolus, there was also a little tenderness in one, sometimes both, calves. In many cases, the patient would remember that there had been a little pain, a little soreness in the leg, and the chart would show a slight temperature rise a few days before.

These were suggestive signs that anyone could see, nurse, intern, even the patient himself. Along with them went a sign first described by famed blood-vessel surgeon John Homans, of Boston. Flexion of the foot at the ankle, pushing it upward toward the head, causes a contraction of the calf muscles, placing pressure on the deep veins of the calf. And in patients who had had the premonitory signs of trouble, this pressure on the foot caused pain.

Now when surgeons studied the post mortem examinations of fatal cases of pulmonary embolism, with the leg veins as a possible source of the clot always in mind, they discovered the real offender. Deep in the two to four deep veins of the lower leg they found loose clots, lying there without much inflammation, if any, to tie them to the walls of the veins and prevent their floating off in the circulation. From these veins came the marauders that traveled through the circulation. Lying doggo there, they waited for a chance to strike at the lungs.

The explanation of clot formation seemed reasonable, too. The return of blood from the lower leg depends largely on the pressure of muscles, in ordinary use, on the thin-walled veins. But patients were usually kept very quiet following operations; often they lay passive in bed for days with little, if any, movement of the legs. What better situation for the formation of stagnant pools of blood in the veins, favoring clot formation? The same thing happened with patients recovering from any long, debilitating illness, and the incidence of pulmonary embolism in these patients was just about as high as it was in operative cases.

The next step was clear: to prevent those clots from reaching the lung. The treatment, too, was simple. Cut across the passageway itself, so the clots could no longer break off and enter the general circulation. An operation was developed. At first it looked very drastic, for it consisted of making an incision in the upper thigh over the great veins from the leg as they coursed just beneath the fascia lata, the heavy tissue that covers the muscles. Fortunately, the veins were relatively easy to get to there in the passage called Hunter's Canal. The vein was picked up, two heavy ligatures were placed around it, and then it was cut in two. That was important, too, for cutting the vein broke up some of the nerve pathways that caused blood-vessel spasm. And cutting the vein stopped all possibility of passage of the leg-vein clots to the lungs.

Strangely enough, cutting these great veins interfered but little with the circulation of the legs. Blood-vessel surgeons had long recognized that here, as almost everywhere else, the body kept in reserve several times the usable vein area actually involved in carrying the blood. With one main channel blocked, others opened up and by-passed the blood with little interference. Surgeons skilled in blood-vessel surgery need only the knowledge of the presence of clots in the calf veins, as evidenced by fever, a little pain, and a positive Homan's sign, to go ahead and operate; but others, perhaps less certain, could not always be sure. So another test had to be devised. This, too, was simple, a method of actually seeing the clots by taking X-rays of the vein.

This new technique of "venography" or "phlebography" followed the discovery of a set of chemical substances that could be injected into the circulation and that would cast a shadow in the X-ray. (They have been used for years to show up the kidneys. Injected into the arm veins, they travel through the circulation and are poured out in the normal secretions of the kidneys, where the X-ray shows them up with a pattern of the inside of the kidneys.)

Blood-vessel surgeons tried injecting these chemicals into leg veins and taking an X-ray picture while the solution was still inside them. It was not a new idea; heart students had used it to show the inside of the heart. Complete pictures of the leg veins are obtained in this way, and surgeons studying those pictures can see where a clot interferes with the proper filling of a deep vein, indubitable evidence of the presence of the potential lung embolus. With this evidence they can proceed without hesitation to tie off the vein above the clot. When this operation was first adopted only a few years ago, deaths from lung embolus took an appreciable drop.

Sometimes even now the clot is not discovered until it has progressed beyond the leg. Again, particularly in infection of the great pelvic vein channels deep in the body, such as happens in postchildbirth and similar conditions, the clots fill the vein channels right up to where they join to form the great single-track vein through the trunk, the vena cava.

These cases are particularly dangerous, for many of them result in fatal embolus attacks. The method of stopping them, too, was easy to see: tie off the vena cava itself, along with a couple of small veins on either side. There'd be no way then for the clots to escape. But that meant tying off the main blood return route from both legs, an unheard of procedure ten years ago. What would happen if the main blood route were thus interrupted?

Doctors fell back on the adage they had used in the leg veins, that usually there were more than enough potential blood channels to compensate for a block in any main channel. Veins were known deep around the spine that could carry the blood, others traveled through the abdominal wall; everywhere there was a vast network of possible detours. So gynecologists treating these infections put their courage in their hands and tied off the vena cava above the involved organs.

First published results came from Tulane University, in New Orleans, where pioneer vascular surgeon Alton Ochsner and his associates developed the knowledge of blood-vessel surgery to a high point. They were amazingly successful. The vena cava could be tied off—surgically, it was relatively easy to reach—blood did by-pass it effectively, and embolus was averted. This was a tremendous victory over surgery's all-powerful enemy, embolism.

A few cases will always occur; some still come absolutely without warning. But many can be prevented by heparin and Dicoumarin, the anti-blood-clotting substances, which are now freely available. In fact, there is much evidence that the incidence of embolism can be substantially reduced merely by administering these drugs in cases known from previous experience to be liable to its occurrence. It may be that anti-coagulant drugs will completely replace surgery for the prevention of fatal lung-clot catastrophe. At present, medical knowledge of this aspect of the embolus problem is not complete enough to allow a final statement. It is enough to say that in surgery of the leg vein, in the powerful anti-clot, thrombus-preventing drugs, surgeons possess a weapon that has almost driven the enemy from the field.

This accomplishment alone would seem to be enough cause for satisfaction to justify surgeons in resting on their laurels. But the medical profession is dedicated to the principle of striving eternally to put itself out of business—by preventing disease. So a new principle has been developed to keep the blood moving in the legs and keep it from slowing down long enough to form a potential embolus clot.

We know now that patients need no longer be kept in bed over long periods. Operative cases are got out of bed now in a day or two; sometimes, with hardy individuals, on the day of operation. Further, it is recognized that even in heart disease, early ambulation is of value, shattering all previous concepts of treatment. With patients up and about at an early period after operation, vein complications decrease rapidly, and lung complications also tend to disappear. And strangely enough, abdominal distension and nausea are also materially diminished.

So striking have been the results of getting patients out of bed almost from the moment they leave the operating table that it has spread to other fields of surgery. Now even brain-injury cases literally wake up and walk.

15.

WAKE UP AND WALK

===

> *Brain surgery—Types of skull injuries—The spine*
> *and the meninges—Operations for hemorrhage*
> *inside the skull—Blood pressure in brain trou-*
> *bles—Spinal puncture—Treatment by dehydra-*
> *tion—Open head wounds no longer fatal—Early*
> *ambulation in head injuries*

Injuries involving the skull and brain have rightly been regarded with fear since ancient times. Evidence of the importance attached to such injuries is found in the crude instruments with which primitive man sought to trephine the skull, instinctively attempting to combat the increase in pressure that practically always follows severe injury to the head. Even in Egyptian papyri, the oldest medical records, is found evidence that those ancient physicians sometimes became very skilled in drilling the skull and often, no doubt, actually relieved symptoms and perhaps saved lives endangered by the accumulation of blood clots inside the skull, which medical men call "hematomata."

In World War I the first great steps toward standardizing methods of handling wartime injuries to the skull and brain were taken when famed neurosurgeon, Dr. Harvey Cushing, demonstrated the feasibility of treating brain injuries very much as the neurosurgeon treats any other condition in his highly specialized field, by meticulous surgery performed by acknowledged specialists. Dr. Cushing demonstrated beyond possibility of doubt that surgery had much to offer the brain wound, and that the principles governing treatment of any wound applied equally well to injuries of that most vital of all organs, the brain.

To understand how surgery is making damaged brains whole again, whether in victims of shell fire or industrial or automobile accidents, a word or two about the nervous system. The great center of control for all body functions, the nervous system is divided into the central and peripheral divisions.

The central nervous system comprises the brain, essentially composed of an upper portion, the cerebrum, where the thought processes, the conscious and subconscious functions, are located; the cerebellum, which controls position and equilibrium; and the medulla, which tapers into the great nerve tract running down the bony canal formed by the front portions of the vertebrae of the spinal column, called the spinal canal.

Encased within the bony box we call the skull, the brain is protected from external violence, and within the spinal canal, the spinal cord is equally well protected. Such protection is needed, for both are extremely vulnerable to any external force.

Injure the brain, remove the portion controlling a section of the body, and loss of function in that region results. Injure the occipital lobes at the back of the brain, where the centers for vision are located, and disturbances in that vital function will occur. Damage the temporal lobes opposite the section of the skull we know as the temple, and defects in hearing result. Or again, injure the localized portion of the cerebrum where originates motor control of the arms and legs and paralyses result. A surprising number of fractured-skull cases lose their sense of smell from injury to the tapering olfactory lobes just back of the eye sockets.

In the lower portion of the brain are located the really vital centers, for here are the tiny concentrations of highly specialized nerve tissue that govern such vital functions as respiration and circulation. For this reason injuries to the base of the skull are the most dangerous of all.

No centers are located in the spinal cord proper, but through it pass the great nerve trunks to every other part of the body. A broken or slipped vertebra, shearing down upon the spinal cord, may shut off all function below the area of injury. Fractures of the neck are often fatal, because with them goes paralysis of the muscles carrying on the vital function of respiration.

Doctors insist on careful handling for cases involving injury to the spinal cord. Needless jack-knifing of an injured back may mean pressure on an uninjured or only slightly damaged spinal cord, increasing many times the injury already present. Medical soldiers are taught to evacuate these patients face-down on the stretcher, with blankets folded under the upper chest and pelvis, preserving the normal curvature of the spine and tending to remove any pressure that may be acting on the nerve trunks of the spinal cord.

Sometimes injury to the back causes only the formation of blood clots inside the unyielding canal of the spinal column. These then press on the vulnerable nerve trunks and cause the same symptoms as an actual injury from slipping bone. Here is the place where the neurosurgeon must dissect deep into the muscles around the spine to expose the roof of the bony canal, the lamina, and cut away a window through which he can inspect the injury and remove the clot. This operation of "laminectomy" is a valuable one also where an uncorrectable vertebral injury is pressing on the spinal cord. Removal of the bony roof over the injured area will often allow complete function to appear when the body seems irrevocably paralyzed below the point of new pressure.

The same bony covering that protects the brain from external violence also constitutes a potential hazard. Injury to the skull may be of two types, and neurosurgeons outline their treatment according to the class into which a particular injury falls.

First are closed injuries, so called because though the skull may be cracked, sometimes by many radiating fractures, just as an eggshell may crack along a dozen radiating lines when struck on one side, there is actually no opening through which the brain is exposed. These are the common injuries of civilian life, in automobile accidents, in barroom brawls, and from such prosaic occurrences as slipping in the bathtub. They constitute by far the largest group of head injuries, both in civilian and military surgery, and books have been written about the mechanism of injury and the treatment best suited to individual cases.

The second great group of cases includes the open injuries, those in which a portion of skull is torn away by direct violence or by a projectile, such as a shell fragment or a bullet. The variety of such accidents is amazing. Every anatomical-curiosity museum contains at least one skull picture exhibiting injuries incredibly severe but which the recipients survived. Classic is one familiar to every medical student in which an iron crowbar was driven completely through the frontal portion of the skull, causing very little damage.

The frontal lobes of the brain, more than any others, are expendable, a fact that accounts for a brand-new subscience called "psychosurgery," by which the surgeon's knife actually cures the one illness that doctors thought would never be treated successfully by the scalpel, insanity.

A closed injury of the skull without fracture is called concussion, but usually, even if fracture is present, the injury to the brain is concussion. Concussion is a temporary paralysis of nervous function, that is, unconsciousness. In true concussion there are no actual hemorrhages either around or into the brain, but the injury is confined to a sudden jarring, which disturbs the brain tissue even more than a direct wound.

It is well understood now that when a force is applied to the skull, such as an attacker's blackjack or a beer bottle, the brain is suddenly set in motion, that is, accelerated. Investigators have even figured out the rate of acceleration that must occur to cause unconsciousness. Coupled with this phenomenon of acceleration is the impact of the moving brain against the other side of the skull, described by the French word *contrecoup*.

Every surgeon is familiar with the picture of a brain underneath a severe head wound, with no injury evident, but fatally compressed on the opposite side by hemorrhage from blood vessels ruptured by the *contrecoup* injury. All this makes it important that the surgeon who treats a head injury not only be thoroughly familiar with the anatomical construction of the brain but also understand the physiological disturbances of function that may follow these injuries.

A famous American anatomist always gave a lecture to

his students on "The Skull as a Closed Box." This concept, more than any other single fact in the history of neurosurgery, has helped doctors understand the problems of head injuries. For the skull, to all intents and purposes, is a closed box of bone containing the brain. Of course this bony helmet was developed because the brain, more than any other part of the body, needs protection at all times. But even while protecting, the unyielding cranium constitutes the brain's most dangerous liability, since it makes the delicate nerve tissue all the more vulnerable to internal disturbances. Concussion, hemorrhage, anything that damages the brain, is usually followed by swelling. All injured tissues swell, but brain swelling occurs in a closed space. Something has to give way if the swelling continues.

If we consider the brain as a tissue that is only moderately compressible, surrounded by two variable factors, the blood it contains and the spinal fluid that surrounds it and fills the ventricles inside the brain, we have a picture of the contents of the skull. The spinal fluid is formed inside the brain in one of the four central cavities, called ventricles. It escapes through several open spaces into the area between the brain and the inside of the skull. If anything interferes with the escape of this fluid—or its absorption back into the blood stream through microscopic projections from the lining membranes, the meninges—the spinal-fluid volume increases.

A prenatal defect in the proper control of the spinal fluid results in monstrosities called hydrocephalics, children with heads swollen into horrible travesties of a normal child's skull. Fortunately, they rarely survive birth. For a long time brain surgeons were powerless to aid even the less severe cases, but under the leadership of the late Baltimore surgeon, Dr. Walter Dandy, an operation was devised to control the rate of formation of the fluid, preventing to a large degree its accumulation under pressure.

The amount of spinal fluid does not ordinarily change much in closed skull injuries. Two other things may occur, however, either one dangerous, often fatal. One is hemorrhage, free bleeding from a torn blood vessel as it passes from the bony wall of the skull to the meninges. These hemorrhages tend to accumulate in one of two positions. Between the skull and meninges around the brain, they are called "extradural" hemorrhages because they are outside the dura mater, the tough outer layer that surrounds the brain. The other position is between the dura mater and the brain, enclosed within the space in which the spinal fluid circulates. Here they are liable to develop more slowly, often they are insidious and are not discovered for a long time, if at all, until the patient begins to complain of continued headaches or show some of the localizing signs familiar to the trained neurosurgeon. Only in comparatively recent times have surgeons realized that many sequelae of brain injuries are due to these strange accumulations of blood, which we group under the term "subdural hematoma." Realizing this, surgeons are quicker now to attack them.

More dangerous, because it is more rapid, is the collection of blood between the skull and the meninges, usually due to rupture of one of the branches of the tiny middle meningeal artery, which branches out here on each side of the skull. In a patient developing an extradural hemorrhage, the symptoms often develop with dramatic suddenness. Only by alert recognition of these symptoms, often tipped off by the seemingly inconspicuous sign of a dilated eye pupil on the side of the injury, can surgeons hope to save many of these patients.

Operation is indicated in extradural hemorrhage, rapid operation by drilling through the skull with a bone-cutting instrument familiar to surgeons as a "Hudson Burr." The surgeon searches for the bleeding, and when he finds it, enlarges the window in the skull until the pressing clot can be removed and the bleeding vessel stopped. Often only the heroic measure of compressing the middle meningeal artery where it actually passes through the bone of the skull will control these hemorrhages. No other operation yields such dramatic dividends as a successful exploration of this kind.

But not every head injury develops a hemorrhage to the point of clot formation; in fact, only a relatively small portion of them do. More usual is an immediate loss of consciousness, lasting for varying periods of time. Often the severity of the injury can be pretty definitely determined from the duration of unconsciousness. Following this is a period of increased pressure from swelling of the brain. It is this cerebral edema that the doctors sometimes find hard to handle. For a while brain surgeons thought they had the answer in an operation whereby an opening was made into the skull to relieve the pressure and give the swelling brain room to expand. But experience has proved the fallacy of this idea and now, although surgeons are drilling burr holes with increasing frequency to hunt for possible blood clots pressing on the brain, the operation of "subtemporal decompression," as it was called, has largely been abandoned.

Surgeons now attack the closed brain injury more intelligently, keeping in mind the facts of closed-box-skull physiology. They know that when the brain swells two things happen. First, the pressure of the spinal fluid is increased but the amount generally stays about the same. And second, the amount of blood in the skull, which means inside and immediately around the brain, must decrease.

The brain needs a plentiful blood supply, however, particularly the vital centers of circulation and respiration in the medulla. So the first thing the brain does when swelling interferes with the amount of blood flowing in and out of the closed skull, is to raise the blood pressure. As the swelling goes on, the blood pressure will go higher and higher, until finally even the elevated pressure can no longer force an adequate supply through the compressed blood vessels of the brain and the centers begin to fail. They fail first, because they are the most sensitive of all the specialized brain cells. Surgeons long ago learned to use this rising blood pressure as a danger signal to tell them when a patient is suffering from swelling of the brain. Every doctor is familiar with the classic picture of severe brain injury: the slow breathing, the increased blood pressure, the deepening coma of interference with brain circulation.

Three methods of handling brain swelling come to mind. One is breaking the continuity of the closed box of the skull, giving the brain more room to expand and allowing more blood to flow. That was the idea of subtemporal decompression, but it wasn't radical enough unless the surgeon could take away nearly half of the skull, an operation whose very magnitude forbade its use. Through the ordinary operative opening, the brain merely protrudes, sealing itself off by pressure against the bony edges, and little is accomplished.

The second method is to attack the next most easily accessible substance within the skull, the spinal fluid forming a liquid cushion around the brain. Fortunately, the spinal fluid is easy to reach, for it circulates around the spinal cord through the entire spinal canal. So surgeons attack increased pressure by spinal puncture, putting slender needles into the back, slipping them between the vertebrae and entering the space around the spinal cord formed by the meningeal layers. Measurements of this fluid indicate the amount of the pressure, and they draw off the fluid slowly, not all at once but by frequent punctures to remove it as it forms. Probably nothing else has contributed so much to control the effects of closed-head injuries as this method of releasing pressure by tapping the spinal cord.

But there is still another method of controlling swelling and pressure; this is by preventing the swelling. Substances used for this purpose are called dehydrating agents and work in several ways. One, magnesium sulphate, ordinarily called epsom salt, tries to purge the body of fluid and in that way drain it away from the brain. With this method of brain dehydration, the fluid intake is limited sharply so that the available supply of liquid with which swelling may occur is decreased.

Still another method, and probably the most effective of the dehydration measures, is the injection into the blood stream of substances that pull fluid into the circulation, away from the brain tissues. Most frequently used of all these is probably a 50 per cent solution of pure sugar, glucose.

Glucose, like all the other blood-stream drying agents, takes advantage of the fact that many substances, when placed on one side of a membrane like the wall of a blood vessel, tend to absorb water until the concentration on both sides is approximately the same, exerting in this way a drawing action that can be measured accurately as "osmotic pressure." A solution of glucose of normal osmotic pressure is about five per cent, so a solution ten times that strong tends to draw a large amount of water into the circulation, dehydrating the tissues. Every brain surgeon is familiar with this action, and frequently uses it during an operation for brain tumor, when the pressure inside the brain interferes with the removal of the growth.

Other substances besides glucose have been used for brain shrinking. For a while another sugar, sucrose, gained favor. Lately, however, a new method of brain dehydration has come into use which promises to supplant all others. Brain cases, like any injury, suffer from shock and shock can be measured by the disappearance of proteins from the blood stream. Surgeons now treat shock by injecting plasma, the protein-containing portion of the blood, or albumen, the main protein fragment of the plasma. This use of hyperconcentrated plasma or albumen solutions in brain dehydration works going and coming, bringing water from the brain and keeping it from going back again.

Conservative brain surgeons now treat closed-head injuries according to a pattern. They keep the patient at rest, using sedatives if necessary. That's important, for a delirious patient thrashes around and may do himself a great deal of harm. They give an average amount of fluid, but they dehydrate the brain by giving concentrated plasma, glucose, or albumen. And they do spinal punctures at frequent intervals, once or twice a day, until the spinal-fluid pressure is normal, indicating that brain swelling has subsided. Along with these, surgeons maintain a constant watchfulness for any sign of a hemorrhage accumulating inside the skull. If signs develop, they quickly put Burr holes through the bony covering and seek for the clot, removing it through soft rubber tubes and a suction machine, and enlarging the opening to allow control of the bleeding vessel if necessary.

Open-head wounds, those in which the skull is actually open, are not nearly so crippling as is generally thought. The percentage of men able to live normally and even to return to military duty after wounds involving brain penetration, is surprisingly high. British surgeon, Major P. B. Ashcroft, working with a mobile neurosurgical unit in the Middle East, treated and followed more than five hundred cases during World War II. Of those with an injury severe enough to penetrate the skull bone and also the dura mater, the tough, fibrous membrane protecting the brain, only fifteen per cent died; more than half returned to duty. This was in spite of the fact that patients were not always received immediately after wounding. A new principle was thus demonstrated, namely that surgery can be delayed perhaps longer in brain cases than in almost any other type of wound, provided the patient is fortified with plenty of antibiotic drugs to control infection and blood plasma to control shock.

In the actual surgical treatment of brain injuries, a number of peculiarities of nervous tissue must be constantly kept in mind. Surgery of the brain must be delicate, that is an axiom, for damage to brain tissue is permanent. The brain's powers of regeneration are nil. So a surgeon must not blindly search through the brain for foreign bodies, pieces of shrapnel, or most important of all, slivers of bone from the skull driven into the brain tissues. Thorough X-ray examination is important, which is just another way of saying that final treatment should be carried out only when complete facilities are available, of which the skill of the surgeon is only one in a group of important factors.

There is another axiom in head injuries, a principle postulated by famed Boston neurosurgeon Cushing in World War I, namely that "every scalp wound, no matter how trifling, is a potential penetrating wound of the skull." War surgeons don't need to be told this; they see enough of these wounds to recognize its importance. The less well-trained doctor treating accidents is not always equally sage. Nothing is more dangerous for the patient than for the doctor to judge a scalp laceration as simply that and suture it, bottling up infection from a sliver of glass or a piece of the skull driven down into the brain, almost inevitably exposing the patient to that most dreaded of all brain-surgery complications, brain abscess.

Nursing care of the brain injury is always important, yet another reason for handling these cases only at base hospitals, where the rush of emergency is not so great. Delirious patients must be sedated and kept from injuring themselves. Infections must be treated with antibiotic drugs, with transfusions.

Most dramatic of all, however, is the new way of handling these convalescent patients, a method more widely used every day for cases of concussion. Ten years ago, the patient with a severe head wound was kept in bed for weeks after operation. In many hospitals, a concussion with perhaps a fifteen-minute period of unconsciousness meant three weeks in bed afterward.

Early in the first of those great battles of the air, the Battle of Britain, the British found that they didn't have room to keep head injuries in bed for weeks. So they had to let them up early, sometimes in a matter of hours after the injury occurred. Thus men with head injuries literally did "wake up and walk." British surgeons fully expected complications, an increased incidence of that puzzling set of symptoms doctors label "postconcussion syndrome."

What happened was hardly believable. These men who had been knocked out for fifteen minutes, even an hour or so, and those who had simple fractures of the skull, woke from their stupor, and with a little encouragement, walked. Not only did they walk, but in many instances their symptoms evaporated practically overnight. They didn't have headaches, they were able to go to meals, and in a few days could go back to their homes. This was a miracle that many medical men still can't believe, and one that is quite difficult to explain.

Working from this observation, the British began to let their head-wound patients get up, too. As soon as they have recovered from the operation and show that they are not going to develop a dangerous infection, patients are now allowed out of bed. A few days later they begin normal activities. Of course they begin with light duties, but they are encouraged to use their hands, to recover lost skills, and to get out and socialize with other patients. In a busy ward there are plenty of light jobs besides the much maligned K.P., and these men are set to doing them. Occupational therapy like this has proved tremendously effective.

It was a daring concept, this idea of letting damaged brains wake up and walk, but it is paying dividends every day. Neurosurgery is a growing infant science of surgery. The succeeding chapters tell more of its development.

16.

PSYCHOSURGERY

Removal of frontal lobe of brain, effects on mental illness—Severing of pathways from frontal lobe—Moniz' operation—American variations—Resulting personality changes—Mental illnesses in which surgery is not indicated—The future of psychosurgery

Since ancient times man has sought for some material explanation for mental disease. Naturally it was simpler to conclude that the sharp mental changes that could turn an alert human into little more than a vegetating mass of protoplasm must have some basis in tangible change in the brain tissues, some tumor growth or degeneration of cells that could be pointed out as the offending area and that might lend itself to surgical approach.

Sometimes, it is true, mental change does follow damage to portions of the brain. One of the earliest recorded medical writings, the Edwin Smith papyrus, demonstrates that the ancient Egyptians realized that mental change often followed injury to the frontal lobes of the brain, the portion occupying the forward part of the skull. It is even reported that these Egyptian psychiatrists, if you can call them such, advised "verbal therapy," the earliest known forerunner of psychoanalysis.

The Greek concept of the uterus as a wandering organ causing mental disturbances gave us the name for one of the commonest and in many ways the most startling types of mental illness, hysteria. In their efforts to treat this strange disease, whereby whole sections of the body may become

171

paralyzed and insensible in a second or total blindness and deafness may appear and disappear with equal facility, the reproductive organs were sacrificed many times by ambitious early surgeons.

Later, with surgery made safer by the discoveries of Pasteur and Lister, surgeons operated boldly on other organs, removing the appendix, tonsils, gall bladder, even the colon, with a view to relieving mental disease. Strangely enough these operations appeared to work in some cases, lending credence to the surgeons' claims. Now we know that the effects were not from the operation but from the shock that attended it. Useful as a physical basis for mental-disease treatment, shock has been popularized largely in insulin, metrazol, and electric-shock treatment.

In the latter part of the nineteenth century German surgeons carried the idea of treating mental disease by operation even further. They removed the portion of the brain governing the particular function most disturbed by the mental disease under treatment. Hallucinations of hearing, common in such types of insanity as dementia praecox, were treated by removing the portions of brain beneath the temples, the temporal lobes of the cerebrum, and beneficial results were claimed. As early as 1910, the nerve fibers between the frontal and parietal lobes of the brain had been cut, an operation similar in many ways to the one now performed with considerable success in the treatment of selected cases of mental illness.

Brain surgeons have long noted that whenever it becomes necessary to remove large portions of the frontal lobes of the brain from normal individuals, because of injury or tumor, a peculiar change in their mental make-up takes place. Essentially it is almost as if a restricting element in the brain has been removed, and the entire personality of the individual often changes. He may become suddenly quite happy-go-lucky, even a little "wacky," his behavior marked by a lack of restraint foreign to him before the operation.

Neurologists had noted that when chimpanzees were given test performances to carry out, making mistakes often produced in them very much the same reaction that occurs in the normal human being—irritation, restlessness, the general picture that mental specialists call neurotic behavior. If these same animals then underwent removal of the frontal lobes of the brain, their reaction to mistakes changed entirely. No longer did they show the pattern of neurotic behavior described in 1935 by neurologist Carlyle Jacobsen. Instead, the response was more nearly what might be characterized as a "don't give a damn" attitude.

This was about the state of our knowledge of the effect of surgical procedures on mental behavior by 1935. It was generally conceded that the frontal lobes of the brain, probably by means of special tracts of nerve fibers connecting them with other portions of the cerebrum located in the most posterior portions of the skull, exerted an inhibiting and balancing effect on mental processes. In a way they acted as a counterbalance of sobriety and thoughtfulness, keeping in check the more unrestrained mental reaction taking place in other sections of the brain.

Sometimes, in line with these concepts, the balance swung too far and the frontal lobes assumed preponderance. Then there occurred types of mental disease characterized by marked depression, those strange guilt urges that keep people washing their hands all day long to remove imaginary stains. These are classified by psychiatrists as "obsessive-compulsive neuroses." Or the melancholic states associated with the "change of life" in both males and females—in short, conditions in which the restraining phases of mental activity predominate to the exclusion of normal mental balance.

Brain surgeons already knew how these symptoms could be controlled in many cases, for sometimes these patients developed tumors or injuries, requiring removal of large portions of the frontal lobes of the brain. Operation often produced a marked change, just as it had in Dr. Jacobsen's chimpanzees. But removal of the frontal lobes was a serious operation, not always successful, and not one to be carried out merely because it might help mental disease.

Then there occurred in 1935 the Second International Neurological Congress in London. Here a neurologist from Portugal, Egas Moniz, presented the novel and interesting concept that since the mental disturbances noted were thought to result from an abnormal preponderance of the frontal lobes over the remainder of the brain, and since it was known that the connections between these frontal lobes and the rest of the brain lay in certain tracts, called "association pathways," to the frontal lobe, severing these pathways should have very much the same effect as removing the lobes themselves. Continuing this line of thought, Moniz had even devised a method of severing the pathways, and reported some success.

Moniz' operation depended on the sensitivity of nerve cells to damage. It is true all over the body that wherever a cell becomes highly specialized, it loses much of its protection against noxious influences, such as the toxins produced by bacteria, or chemical poisons, and most important, its resistance to lack of oxygen is markedly decreased. Brain cells are some of the most highly specialized in the entire body and are most susceptible to injury. Lack of oxygen will kill them quite quickly, although other body cells may continue to live for some hours in nearly complete absence of oxygen.

Moniz and his surgical colleague, Lima, worked out an ingenious way of damaging the nerve-fiber pathways to the frontal lobes of the brain. First, they made a small incision in the scalp on either side of the midline and just in front of the line drawn across the skull at the level of the ears. A small trephine opening was then made through the skull bone, exposing the brain. By inserting a needle here and injecting alcohol, they were able to injure the nerve pathways to the frontal lobes, because brain cells are abnormally sensitive to direct injection of alcohol.

Alcohol injections soon proved not quite sufficient to accomplish their intentions, so Moniz and Lima shortly changed their technique. They began to use a blunt needle, which was passed from side to side through brain tissue to cut across the nerve fibers to the frontal lobes. The trick here was to break the nerve pathways but not damage any blood vessels that might cause a hemorrhage into the brain, leading to paralysis and similar undesirable occurrences.

Other surgeons, notably Walter J. Freeman and James W. Watts, American pioneers in this type of operation, James G. Lyerly, and others, have modeled their operations somewhat after the original principle of Moniz. Generally, the procedure is simple. The patient's head is shaved and some type of basal anesthetic is given to make him drowsy on the morning of the operation. Novocain is injected into the areas marked out for the trephine openings, and small incisions, barely an inch long, are made through the scalp. An ingenious trephine is used to extract a button of bone from the skull; this is replaced after the operation and heals back into place.

With the brain exposed through these small openings, instruments are inserted into the brain and moved across the nerve pathways to the frontal lobes, severing the association nerve fibers. The wound is inspected carefully then for bleeding, the bone button replaced, and a few stitches bring the skin together. As far as the patient is concerned, the operation doesn't amount to nearly the discomfort of a tonsilectomy.

A different form of this operation has been used in more recent years but has never been generally popular with surgeons performing psychosurgery. Instead of drilling a hole into the skull, a needle is passed through the upper wall of the eye socket, where the bone is quite thin, and the association fibers are disrupted from below.

Following operation, these brain-sectioned patients show very interesting effects almost immediately. There may be some headache for a few days, although many patients refuse to believe that they have had an operation. Vomiting may last as long as two to four days. The patient is usually in a state of apathy, lying quietly and serenely in bed. In a person intensely agitated and anxious before operation, this sudden change in demeanor following such a simple procedure is miraculous, to say the least. The somnolence persists for perhaps a week after operation, then disappears, although some patients remain somewhat apathetic for many weeks.

It is not surprising that patients who have had "prefrontal lobotomy," the name given to this operation, are confused for a while, considering the profound changes in the brain. This soon passes off, however. A few are restless and definitely euphoric. One patient, seen in the early days of this procedure, was so depressed before operation that tube feeding was required and suicide had been attempted. On the morning after the operation he was laughing and singing, the complete reverse of his former apathy.

Most striking of all, however, is the change in the patients' mental outlook. Sometimes they are remarkably frank and tend to speak out without hesitation on subjects they normally might not mention. Especially are they liable to interject their opinions, whether asked for or not, into subjects under discussion. Nor are they intentionally critical, for they often recognize almost immediately that their comment had perhaps better have been left unsaid, and apologize for their thoughtlessness. At the same time there is no tendency to morbid introspection such as characterized their thinking before.

Lack of initiative is said to be characteristic of the prefrontal-lobotomy patient. Sometimes this goes on to actual dullness and deterioration, but more often it is a diminution in the drive that, before operation, may have been so marked as to lead to overactivity. The operation does not usually affect the intelligence. Sometimes more accuracy is noted because the sick person is free from worry for the first time since the onset of his illness.

Perhaps the most characteristic result of prefrontal lobotomy is a marked lessening of the individual's abstraction with self, manifested by renewed interest and identification with the world around him. It might almost be said that the operation changes an introvert into an extrovert, although this is not strictly true. Patients with marked introvertive tendencies may retain them after operation, but there is less effect from introvertive thinking, less tendency toward morbidness and preoccupation with one's own mental processes.

A most constant symptom in many mental diseases is a preoccupation with the bodily functions. To most of us, the normal functioning of our digestive and eliminative systems is a matter of no particular concern; the organs are there, governed by their own automatic or autonomic nervous system. Their function is taken as a matter of course and no attention is paid to them unless some abnormality presents itself.

To the mentally ill person these normal physiologic processes cause intense mental preoccupation. Their complaint is endlessly that of trouble with the stomach, the head, and almost any portion of the body. Prefrontal lobotomy tends to relieve this preoccupation and to cut the emotions loose from such automatic body processes. The patient may still be conscious of his stomach and his head, but it troubles him little or not at all, still further evidence that the change is essentially to "Don't give a damn."

Just why these changes take place after a simple operation like prefrontal lobotomy has aroused considerable interest in brain surgeons and neurologists. Its effects are not explainable simply on the basis of the interruption of nerve tracts, for exactly the same results may follow shock treatment or even, in some cases, psychoanalysis alone. Most neurologists think that much of the effect of the operation results from a severance between the brain cortex, which governs the major processes involved in emotional feeling, and the brain nuclei which act as centers for such aspects of the thought processes.

Not all mental disease lends itself to successful treatment by prefrontal lobotomy. In some cases it is definitely contraindicated. For instance, in a form of insanity recurring in cycles and called "manic depressive psychosis," the patient goes alternately from periods of deep depression, in which he may do himself bodily harm by attempts at suicide, to periods of mania, in which he may become actually destructive. To operate on such a case in the stage of depression may mean an apparent return to normal in a few days, following which, as if the other side of the balance wheel had been removed, the mania may return and be much worse, perhaps making it necessary to restrain the sick man to prevent his harming others and himself in the exuberance of his good feeling.

That there is a great place for this operation most psychosurgeons agree, as well as many psychiatrists.

Decision to operate is based not so much on the actual type of mental disease as on the symptoms. Generally speaking, those who respond best are minds preoccupied with depressive thoughts to the point of exclusion of almost every normal impulse and emotion. Most characteristic of these are the "affective psychoses," which include the so-called "involutional depressions" occurring with the change of life, and "agitated depressions" during middle age. Good results in as high as 75 per cent of these cases have been reported. Apparently the operation severs the connections between the patient and a conscience that rides herd on him like a true "Old Man of the Sea."

In schizophrenia, split personality, prefrontal lobotomy is successful at times but not as a general rule. The duration of the disease determines somewhat the chances of success. Cases of explosive character, developing in a short time, lend themselves best to treatment, and results are usually fairly good. In widespread mental degeneration, such as that found in true dementia praecox, operation is often futile.

One strange type of mental disturbance is often relieved by prefrontal lobotomy. Interestingly enough, it represents only a slight change from normal mental behavior. Many of us feel a compulsion to check a locked door to see that it is really locked, to smell the gas range to be certain that it is turned off, to wash our hands time and again because we feel some dirt still clings to our fingers. Carry these normal processes a little further and they become obsessions, forcing us to wash our hands endlessly, to perform time and again little acts that are not necessary but that an inner drive to perfectionism will not allow us to stop. These variations from normal are classified as obsessive-compulsive neuroses, and in extreme forms may occupy the individual's every thought and action.

In such obsessive neuroses, prefrontal lobotomy again appears to interrupt the connections between the individual and his hard-riding conscience. The urge seems to be there, but again the patient does not feel the continual drive to assuage the urgings of his conscience.

Some conservative mental specialists shun prefrontal lobotomy. To them the apathy and general "don't give a damn attitude" that often develop after it are as bad as the original illness. An equally large proportion feel that removing the danger of suicide from an obsessed or agitated patient is worth the change in his mental status. The large number of such cases successfully treated and returned to society tends to bear out this optimistic view.

Two new drugs, Reserpine and chloropromazine, seem to hold great promise now of becoming the greatest addition to the psychiatrist's armamentarium in this century. Whether they will displace prefrontal lobotomy and other time-honored methods of treatment remains, of course, to be seen. However, even the first results of their use are so promising that in all probability they will considerably lessen both psychosurgery and convulsive treatment in mental disorders.

17.

IT MAY NOT BE SCIATICA

Causes of sciatica—The sacroiliac joint—The spinal column and hernia of the intervertebral disc—Operation to cure it—Similar ailments, bursitis, neuritis

There is a good bit of the ridiculous in the picture we have come to associate with the unhappy sufferer from sciatic-nerve pain. We see him in cartoons and funny magazines, in advertisements for trick belts and patent medicines, even in the chaste announcements of chiropractors and osteopaths, along with the assurance that this and all other diseases can be cured with only one treatment. Always the picture is the same, the pained expression, the hand resting on the hip, the unnatural angle of the body, as if every movement brought forth indescribable pain, as it often does.

Why such agony should be funny to the onlooker is at first glance hard to see. Yet the patient himself feels a great deal of shame, too, in his recurring disability. Perhaps it is the knowledge that he feels ridiculous that makes the rest of us see him as such. Certainly, to him, it is a matter of shame that at times he cannot bend down to lace his shoes without feeling something snap in his back and an agonizing pain shoot down his leg. Or he squeezes his wife in a burst of conjugal enthusiasm—and is laid up for a week.

This is the picture we have come to associate with the sciatica sufferer, this and the other more realistic picture of the liniment advertisements, the bent leg, the sciatic nerve apparently on fire, sending shooting pains up and down the limb.

Unfortunately, to the doctor the sciatic picture hasn't always been very much clearer. The anatomy of the sacroiliac joint, the double wing-shaped articulation whereby the spine is attached to the pelvic bones, is well known. X-rays, even in the most acute types of strain, rarely demonstrate any disturbance of the joint. No reason for nerve irritation can be shown, yet the patient endures excruciating pain, a couple of feet of his midsection entirely rigid and immovable from spasm of his back muscles. Often he is unable to turn over in bed.

And if the pathology of this affliction was not well known, until recently treatment was not much better. A few days' rest in bed, particularly a firm bed that did not give to the weight of the body, often alleviated the symptoms. Heat, infra-red, short-wave diathermy—all of them gave relief sometimes, but as often had no effect at all. Tight belts seemed to aid more than anything else. Sometimes there was magical relief from novocain injections; as often there was no effect. Operations that slit the fascia, the thick, fibrous band encircling the muscles of the hips and back, seemed to help some cases; as often again, they had no effect whatsoever.

A headache to the doctor, a recurring source of agony and shame to himself, the sciatica sufferer went on his way. At first the pain stayed in the back and hips, then gradually it began to spread down the leg, usually the same one. Soon he noticed that coughing or sneezing sent an excruciating hot flash of pain down to his knee, sometimes down to his heel. He began to lean toward the good leg, unconsciously keeping the weight off the painful one, gradually developing a sort of stiff-backed limp as he sought more and more to favor the painful limb.

This was the picture in many sciatica or "sacroiliac" sufferers after months or years of recurring attacks. Sometimes they would go for months with no symptoms and begin to think they were well. Then some trivial activity, digging in the garden, a swing at golf, the same movement they'd performed a hundred times before, and the pain was back, crippling them for weeks at a time.

A little over a decade ago, a few neurosurgeons and neurologists began to observe critically this question of sciatic-nerve pain. They studied the symptoms and found that a large group of sufferers fell into a pretty characteristic pattern. They could even tell almost exactly which nerve was involved, and in a great proportion of cases it was the same one. Now they were really getting at the problem. It boiled down to the fact that sciatica—not in all cases but still in a respectable percentage—was irritation not of the whole sciatic nerve, which is formed by the junction of about half a dozen separate roots of the nerves coming off the spinal cord near its lower end, but of only one or two of the roots that make up the nerve.

To confirm this localization to single nerve roots, they studied the neurological examinations of these patients and learned still more by tapping, pinpricking, and asking "Sharp or dull?" In a lot of these cases, tapping on the tendon back of the ankle produced no foot jerk. The knee jerk was usually present, but the ankle jerk almost always failed to appear. Here was strong confirmation that the trouble involved the lower portion of the sciatic-nerve roots. When sensation was tested, it, too, was usually changed in the area supplied by one or two nerves, those coming out at the extreme lower end of the spinal column's movable vertebrae, the lumbar spine.

It was simple then to conclude that something had slipped and pressed on the nerves. But what could it be? The vertebrae could be ruled out almost immediately. When they slipped enough to press on nerves, there had usually been a severe injury to the back, and these cases did not have any such injury. Then there were often cases involving the extreme lower portion of the back, in which the fifth lumbar vertebra, the lowest one, did slip forward as much as half to three-quarters of an inch, a condition the orthopedist had long known by the jaw-breaking name of "spondylolisthesis." But these cases rarely got nerve-root pain. Another thing—if pressure of slipped vertebrae was the cause, both legs should be affected, and this was rarely the case.

All the evidence boiled down to the fact that something they couldn't see, even in the X-ray, was pressing on the nerve roots to one leg and causing all this pain, something that varied in its pressure. Sometimes it didn't press at all; at other times the force was great enough to paralyze the nerves.

Spinal-cord tumors could do that, but they didn't change so quickly from normal-to-pain-to-normal-again. The place to go for the answer was where every surgeon goes when he gets stuck. First to the anatomy book and then to the skeleton.

The answer was found in the skeleton. The spinal column is made up of individual bones that sit on top of each other. They are threaded on the spinal cord, the great nerve tract from the brain to the rest of the body, in almost exactly the way a group of boys getting ready for a ball game place hand over hand on the bat to determine the first at the plate. Each individual vertebra is composed of a solid disclike body pointing forward, from which spring two bony arms to form a circle and project in the back as the spines. The circle upon circle of the vertebrae form the spinal, or vertebral, canal in which the spinal cord lies. Between each vertebra and the one above and the one below it, there are tiny joints, called articulations, which give the spinal column its flexibility from side to side.

To obtain flexibility from front to back, a different mechanism is necessary. It is found in the intervertebral discs of cartilage, the elastic gristlelike substance often found at the ends of bones and entering into the formation of joints. Each vertebral body rests on a cushion of soft cartilage, which in turn rests on the body of the next vertebra below it. But even though cartilage is elastic, there wouldn't be much movement if it weren't for another curious fact: the inside of these intervertebral discs is almost liquid, a pulplike substance called the nucleus pulposus and held in place by a more solid rim around the edge of the disc. The softer center portion acts as a cushion, giving much more mobility to the vertebral column.

So far nothing yet explained the strange individual nerve pressure in these special cases of recurring sciatic pain. Again the anatomists found the clue. In some cases something happened to the firm ring of cartilage that surrounds the soft nucleus pulposus. It broke in spots and allowed the soft inner portion to spurt through, protruding like a small white mushroom into the space around the spinal cord and its nerve roots. But that space is only large enough for the nerve tracts, anything else that protrudes into it would have to infringe on the rights of the structures already there, in this instance the nerve roots. -

There was the explanation of nerve-root pain in some of these cases. It took the name of "herniation of the nucleus pulposus" or "hernia of the intervertebral disc." In surgical parlance a hernia is anything that sticks out from where it is supposed to be, so this is distinctly a hernia. Nobody knows exactly why it elects the lower lumbar spine in many cases and why one disc, that between the last lumbar vertebra and the sacrum, the solid, wedge-shaped "sitting-down bone," is involved so much oftener than the others. But it is perfectly certain that in a lot of cases, these mushroomlike protrusions of the nucleus pulposus do cause sciatic pain.

But how explain the sudden disappearance of pain in these cases at times? That did not take long either. Arch the back forward and the space between the vertebrae seems to be widened, often pulling the jellylike disc right back into place and removing the pressure.

But why didn't it press on both sides? Take a look inside the spinal column and the answer is right there, a strong ligament running down the front of the vertebral body through which the pulpy mass of the herniating disc cannot push— so it goes to one side. That explains the single-leg involvement in most cases.

For the first time now, neurosurgeons felt that they had something to offer in the treatment of these intractable cases of sciatic pain, the ones accompanied by loss of the ankle jerk, weakness of the muscles in the painful leg, changes in the skin sensation due to pressure on the nerve roots. For a while it seemed that nearly all cases of sciatica could be explained that way and treated by operation. Then, as evidence massed, it became clear that hernia of the nucleus pulposus did not explain all cases, although some optimistic nerve surgeons went on believing that it explained most cases.

An ingenious examination was devised and perfected by pioneering surgeons. It depends on the fact that a light oily substance containing iodine, called "lipiodol" or simply "iodized oil," when injected into any portion of the body, casts a heavy shadow on the X-ray, which can be easily identified from surrounding bone.

It was a relatively simple procedure to insert a needle into the spine above the suspected bulging disc, inject a small amount of iodized oil into the spinal canal, and watch it flow downward under the X-ray. If it struck a hump at the level where the herniation was expected to be, the case was clinched.

The trick was to get the oil out again, and that wasn't always easy. A lighter oil was then found that worked better and could be removed more easily. Some others used air to outline the spinal canal and took X-rays of the light areas created by the presence of air. This X-ray demonstration of the bulging disc wasn't perfect, but many conservative neurosurgeons would not operate without this final bit of confirmatory evidence. Others, equally conscientious, felt that they could make the diagnosis from neurological examination alone.

But what of treatment? Didn't it take a formidable operation to cut through all that bone and expose the delicate nerves of the spinal cord? Wasn't it dangerous to remove the nucleus pulposus from around the nerve roots, and wouldn't the back be weak from so much loss of bone?

Again the anatomy books gave the answer. Between each circular bony column that rises from the vertebral body to surround the spinal cord, there is a space covered only by a heavy ligament, the ligamentum flavum. If this ligament is trimmed away over the area in which the nucleus pulposus is suspected to have broken through, a little window is created through which the whole area can be examined—without destroying any bone whatsoever. That took away most of the difficulty of the operation right there. From then on it was relatively simple.

The surgeon makes an incision over the lower portion of the spine a few inches long. He pushes the muscles away until the ligamentum flavum is exposed, and then he carefully trims it loose as a flap and lifts it out of the way. The spinal cord and nerve roots lie underneath, and when he pushes them very gently aside he can see the protrusion of the soft, pulpy mass of the nucleus pulposus at the back of the spinal canal, with the nerve root running over it.

A special instrument used by neurosurgeons comes in handy then. It is called a "pituitary rongeur," and is used for digging brain tumors out of very small pockets beneath the brain. With its long neck, this instrument can be inserted through the window in the ligamentum flavum and right into the opening through which the hernia has come. Now it is possible to remove not only the portion projecting into the spinal canal and pressing on the nerve roots, but all the soft pulp that might later be forced out. A small spoonlike instrument is finally used to scoop, or curette, out the entire central portion of the disc, allowing it to collapse then so that the vertebrae rest on each other and the whole area is made stable.

The operation doesn't bother the patient much. He is so glad to be rid of the pain that he is ready to get up and walk in a few days. In selected cases, ones in which the trouble is definitely due to a demonstrable hernia of the soft, pulpy center of the cartilage disc, results are very good. As is always the case with a new procedure, a lot of patients were thought to be pulposus cases when the cause was actually a real neuritis of the nerve roots, pressure from excess bone thrown down in the course of an arthritic infection, or some other known producer of backache.

Orthopedists tend to believe that herniation of the disc is an infrequent cause of sciatic pain; neurosurgeons are almost equally vehement in their belief that it explains many cases and that operation cures a large percentage of them. The answer, as with most new things, lies somewhere between. Meanwhile, when a herniated disc can actually be demonstrated, the relief afforded the sufferer by this simple—for a trained neurosurgeon—operation is well-nigh miraculous.

Further evidence on the side of the neurosurgeons is the fact that many cases of another very troublesome affliction have recently been shown to be due to herniation of discs in another position. This time it is the shoulder and those baffling cases of pain in the lower neck radiating out into the arms that are variously diagnosed as wry neck, bursitis, and neuritis. A certain proportion of these have been definitely shown to be due to protrusion of the nucleus pulposus between the last one or two neck vertebrae, and operation has given magical relief to many of these sufferers already.

A trick back may still be real sciatica. Or then it may not be sciatica at all but pressure on a nerve root by one of those mushroomlike protrusions of cartilage from the intervertebral disc. If it is, there's an operation that will cure, quickly. A competent neurologist and orthopedist can usually tell which it is.

18.

TANTALUM: THE LIVING METAL

Early uses of metal in the body, reactions—Gold, silver, aluminum, magnesium, vanadium, stainless steel—Vitallium for bone plates, skull plates, replacement of bile ducts and arteries—Its limitations—Tantalum molded into thin plates, thin foil, fine wires—Use in nerve surgery, tantalum sutures, foil coverings—Tantalum foil on brain tissues—Replacing defects in bones—Covering hernias with metal plates—Tantalum gauze—Tantalum in plastic surgery

Since ancient times man has sought a substitute for lost human tissue, a material that could be used inside the body to splint fractures, connect torn nerves and blood vessels, and otherwise simulate the properties of living tissue. Each new discovery had some disadvantages, though usually superior to those that had preceded it. Eternally man has sought for the perfect metallic substance for insertion into the body, one that would not insult body tissues but would continue year after year to perform the function for which it was originally planned. Now such a substance has been found, a metal so inert that it seems to become a part of the living tissue in which it is placed. This new substance is tantalum.

Paradoxically, this new metal, so closely identifying itself with living tissues, possesses least of all metals the attributes of life. Years ago the experiments of Dr. George Crile with an "artificial cell" showed that the processes of living closely approximate the development in living tissues of a difference of electrical potential resulting in the passage of an infinitesi-

mally small electric current. Physiologists have long studied
the electric current set up in living muscles and nerves with
the normal functions of human life, have even measured them
with delicate galvanometers. Most classic example of the
measurement of these currents is the electrocardiograph,
whereby the action currents of the heart muscle are photo-
graphed on a moving film, forming the electrocardiographic
tracing.

The main deterrent to successful use of metals in living tissues, before tantalum, has always been the setting up of electric currents between the metals used and the tissue fluids
surrounding them. Because of these currents, and the physical and chemical changes accompanying them, healing of
tissues was almost always interfered with, bones softened and
were eroded away around screw holes, disturbing "foreign-
body reactions" occurred, tending to vitiate the good results
that the surgeon sought.

Almost four hundred years ago Petronius devised a plate
made of gold to repair the defects of cleft palate, and two
hundred years later, the first metal wire was placed around a
fracture. One deterrent in those days, before Lister's famous
discovery of antisepsis, was the tendency for infection to develop around these implanted foreign substances. But toward
the end of the last century, Lister himself was able to an-
nounce the successful wiring of a fractured kneecap.

With the beginning of the present century, Sir William
Arbuthnot Lane, famed British bone surgeon, began to use
metal plates for fixing fractured bones and devised a set of
such plates and bone screws that are still widely used in
treating fractures of the shaft of the long bones of the arm and
leg. Even before Lane, surgeons had inserted a metal nail
into a fractured hip, presaging the modern treatment of this
distressing complication of old age with nails of stainless
steel and other metals.

Always the search was for substances that would cause little, if any, reaction in the body tissues. Silver was first used
and continued in favor for many years because of its relative inertness and ease of handling. However, it also possessed
some disadvantages, notably its softness, its tendency to

break, and the fact that it was rapidly corroded by oxygen in the body.

Aluminum was used as early as 1893 as a plate to cover a defect in the skull left by a wound. Here, probably more than anywhere else, was a need for a suitable metallic substitute for bone. Wounds and infections often result in the loss of portions of the skull, leaving a pulsating soft area after the scalp has healed over. A blow here might seriously damage the brain. In addition there is the tendency of the brain to move toward the opening and protrude through it, interfering with the proper functioning of that vital and extremely delicate organ. Aluminum unfortunately possesses many of the objectionable features of silver.

Magnesium seemed for a while to be the answer, since it is gradually absorbed into the body, thus removing the necessity of operating once again to remove the foreign body.

Then in about 1920 there was a great revival of interest in metal plates for fractured bones and as a replacement for lost bone in the skull and other portions of the body. A steel alloy, vanadium steel, gave some promise and achieved a certain amount of popularity with bone surgeons. Stainless steel was also used rather widely. With them all, still, went the same observations, that they tended to cause irritation and acted generally as foreign bodies. By 1936, Dr. Charles S. Venable and his associates concluded from their experiments that: "All the metals commonly used in surgery were subject to electrolytic activity in body fluids . . . the extent of tissue damage was roughly equivalent to the amount of galvanic action which took place between the metals."

In their researches, Dr. Venable and his co-workers discovered a dental alloy called vitallium, which seemed to be inert in body fluids and nonirritating to body tissue. These properties gave it immediate and widespread popularity. In the years since its discovery, it has been used as bone plates for fractures, as replacement for lost areas of skull to cover defects, as tubes to substitute for bile ducts and arteries, and as communications between blood vessels. Vitallium has proved satisfactory in almost every respect, save a few mechanical features.

Vitallium, being an alloy, cannot be easily molded and is

not capable of being drawn out into very fine wires or very thin flexible foil. A substance like this was badly needed in many ways, but most of all in neurological surgery. Nerve tissue is extraordinarily delicate and sensitive to any foreign substance. Ordinary sutures, no matter how fine, cause some irritation and tend to interfere with the regrowth of cut nerves. Too, in the neighborhood of injured nerves, scar tissue tends to form, interfering greatly with proper healing of damaged nerve trunks.

Something was needed that could be placed around the repaired nerves, but vitallium, the only substance then in use that was inert enough not to cause any reaction in nerve tissue, could not be prepared in such thin sheets and such hairlike strands. Also, vitallium could not be molded at the operating table into plates to replace lost sections of the skull. It was necessary first to cast the plate to the desired contours, then sterilize it and place it in the bony defect of the skull.

In 1922, after a period of trial and error extending back to 1906–1908, when he was working for his Ph. D. at the University of Pennsylvania, Dr. Clarence W. Balke managed to produce a relatively pure form of a rare new metal called tantalum. Most important of all, this bluish-gray metal could be molded into thin plates, even foils, and into extremely fine wires.

Tantalum wasn't exactly a new metal. As early as 1802, it had been found in conjunction with another element, called columbium, in a new black mineral substance. It was almost a hundred years later that Werner von Bolton produced tantalum in wire form for use as a filament in electric light bulbs. The cost was prohibitive, however, and it was replaced by tungsten a short time later. It is interesting that von Bolton is reported to have made small amounts of pure tantalum which were used as surgical and dental instruments.

With Dr. Balke's discovery of a method of obtaining pure tantalum from the original ore—now found in South Dakota and Colorado as well as many other places over the world—it became more than a laboratory curiosity. It was soon discovered that tantalum had certain very valuable properties in the electric field, mainly because it seemed to act as a "valve" to the flow of electric current. In rectifiers and in tubes used in electronics, tantalum occupied a promising place. Scientists agree that its use in electronics materially expedited our war effort.

With the physical properties of tantalum well established, it was inevitable that it should be considered in man's long search for the perfect metal for use inside the body. Chemically, too, it went a long way toward filling the requirements for this perfect substance.

At body temperatures and in body concentrations of acids and alkalis, tantalum appears completely inert chemically. This means that it resists attack by all chemical substances normally present in the body. No corrosion can occur and, most important of all, no currents of electricity are created by its presence in body fluid. Since Dr. Venable had long ago propounded the principle that tissue damage was in general proportional to galvanic action, tantalum promised to be the perfect substance as far as body reaction went.

But vitallium fulfills that criterion, too. What are the advantages of tantalum over it? In general, the surgical advantages of tantalum depend on the fact that it can be rolled into extremely thin, yet stable, sheets, capable of being molded at the operating table to fit a skull defect, and trimmed to the outlines of that defect with a pair of metal shears. Gossamer-thin wires can be spun of tantalum metal, or paper-thin sheets of foil rolled out. These properties make tantalum more useful than vitallium in many ways, yet they also make it inferior.

Tantalum has not yet been formed into strong metallic plates, since it cannot be cast. For this purpose vitallium will probably continue to be the right hand of the bone surgeon. Nor can screws be so well formed of tantalum as of vitallium. Even so, to argue the benefits of one metal over the other is mere quibbling. There is a definite place for both, each widening as surgical technique encompasses the minor problems of utilizing metallic substances in the body.

Tantalum is widely used for nerve surgery in military hospitals, where the large number of nerve injuries increased its importance hundreds fold. Neurosurgeons can operate on injured nerves, which are protected from reaction and damage to healing by the nonirritating properties of tantalum-wire sutures and the ability of the foil wrapped about the nerve repair to prevent scar tissue from interfering with regeneration.

But nerve suture has not been the most dramatic accomplishment of this strangely inert metal. The repair of skull defects has always been a problem to military neurosurgeons. Skull-bone loss does occur in civilian injuries but to no such extent as in battle. Many substances have been used, none of them altogether satisfactory. One method consists in cutting part way through the thickness of the skull beside the defect, then sliding over a split section of bone to heal in place. Another operation removes sections of rib cartilage, the soft, gristly substance forming the so-called floating ribs, and bridges the gap with it. None of these methods is quite satisfactory, although much has been accomplished. With the advent of vitallium, the defects were sometimes measured and new plates cast of the metal and later inserted in the skull.

By 1942, neurosurgeons were seeking to learn how the properties of tantalum could be adapted to closing skull defects. First it was necessary to learn what effect a plate would have on the brain beneath it. Dr. Robert H. Pudenz, working at McGill University Medical School, had shown in experiments on animals that when tantalum foil was placed on the brain, and even into wounds of the brain, it protected the delicate nerve tissue from excessive scarring, hitherto an unpleasant side effect of brain wounds. Also he had shown that when tantalum was placed directly into the brain, the reaction was almost unbelievably small, amazingly different from other metallic substances. From these experiments, it appeared that tantalum could be safely used in direct contact with brain tissue without aftereffect.

Continuing his experiments, Dr. Pudenz actually replaced cranial defects with tantalum plates and used tantalum clips, tiny V shaped pieces of the metal, to control small blood vessels, always before accomplished by silver clips in brain surgery.

The time was ripe for the actual use of tantalum plates in the human being. This occurred in the Army's Walter Reed Hospital in 1942, when Lieutenant Colonel R. G. Spurling successfully covered a skull defect from a wound with a plate of tantalum metal. Since that time reports of such operations have filled medical journals. A definite technique has been worked out for shaping and cutting the plates, one that borrows again from another science, colloid chemistry, and its application in dentistry.

The first step in preparing a tantalum plate is to outline on the scalp the edges of the defect. Dental compound, or one of the hydrocolloids more recently used in making molds, is then gently molded over the depression in the skull. This compound hardens, producing a negative mold of the defect, and from this a positive mold is cast.

Wax is now used to restore the normal contours to the defective skull, as represented by the metal mold, and from this wax model a zinc die is made. A counter die of lead is then also made. The tantalum plate can then be molded between the two dies, an operation that can be carried out in any dental laboratory. A few holes are drilled into the plate and it is ready for sterilizing.

At the operating table the edges of the skull defect are slotted to receive the tantalum plate, which can then be trimmed with shears to the exact outline desired. The sterile plate is put in place and locked in with tiny, triangular "points" of tantalum tapped into the bone. When the scalp is sutured over this region, it is practically impossible to tell that a foreign substance has been inserted into the skull.

Interestingly enough, tantalum foil is often used at the time brain wounds are treated surgically in preparation for the plate to come at a later operation. Laying the foil over the injured brain prevents scarring, and the brain becomes covered with a thin, glistening membrane of tissue growing close to the foil and forming a new covering for the brain. Even infected wounds have been operated on and tantalum plates inserted, with antibiotic drugs controlling the infection. In more than one case, tantalum plates larger than the palm of a man's hand have successfully remained in the human skull.

These uses do not in any sense exhaust the possibilities of this nearly perfect metal. Bone defects are being replaced by tantalum molds in other parts of the body. Weak areas in body cavities, such as large postoperative hernias, may be covered with thin plates of tantalum, sewn directly to the muscles of the abdominal wall around the hernia. Tantalum wire has even been used to lift up the sagging muscles of the face following facial-nerve injury, eradicating the distressing deformity from which these patients suffer.

Work is now in progress to make cloth of tantalum strands for use as surgical dressings, replacing gauze, which is irritating to raw and burned areas. In plastic surgery involving the construction of new tendons from other body tissues, the use of tantalum foil to provide a smooth running groove in which the new tendon may lie, is only now beginning to break the surface of discovery. Everywhere in surgery there are fields for use of this magically inert metal. New discoveries with tantalum should continue to widen its use. Perhaps the greatest of these will eventually be in plastic surgery.

19.

BUNDLING FOR BURNS

Effects of burns—Tannic-acid treatment, now largely abandoned—Shock in severe burns—Plasma—Infection in burns—Surgery and the wonder drugs—New treatment as surgical operations with vaseline gauze and compression—Early skin grafting

Burns have long been one of the most difficult problems taxing the ingenuity of the civilian doctor. When World War II came, it brought a sharp increase in the incidence of burns, both on the battlefields and on the home front. With more people in industrial work, with transportation geared to a higher tempo in an era of excitement and partial hysteria, it was inevitable that accidents should happen on the home front.

On the battlefields, whether on land or sea, a marked increase in the number of burns resulted from modern methods of warfare—increased use of military motor vehicles, with the constant presence of inflammable gasoline in their tanks; armored warfare in which flames might sweep suddenly through a confined space from which men could escape only with difficulty; airplane crashes spraying the plane with inflammable material and often engulfing it in a roaring holocaust of fire; exploding gun turrets, flame throwers, burning oil from torpedoed boats. All these sharply increased the incidence of burns in wartime, but an even greater threat is posed by the Atomic Age. The bombing of Hiroshima and Nagasaki showed the ability of atomic weapons to produce thousands of burned casualties in an instant. Now more than ever before we need to know all there is to know about burns.

Had American doctors not been prepared, the death rate from burns both in civil life and in the armed forces during World War II and the Korean conflict would have been much higher. Fortunately, the groundwork had been done. The simple principles of modern burn treatment had already been formulated, and as one fortunate result of one of the greatest civilian disasters in modern times, the Boston Cocoanut Grove disaster, these principles were widely known throughout the country. It remained only to put into effect a new treatment for burns that had been so effectively demonstrated as superior over all other existing methods, the compression dressing. This might aptly be called, for lack of any other equally descriptive phrase, "bundling for burns."

The scientific principles used that night in the great Massachusetts General Hospital, when screaming and dying burned casualties were pouring into its emergency room in a seemingly never ending stream, were the culmination of many years of study and investigation, discarding that which was extraneous and of no proved value, taking up new things that seemed to offer fresh possibilities, searching always for the essential scientific truth. In short, these were the very methods of combined scientific investigation and clinical observation that have brought American medicine to its present high knowledge and proficiency in that greatest of all skilled trades —the job of saving lives.

It all began years ago, at least a hundred years ago and perhaps even as far back as any intelligent medical thought existed, which would put it back to that amazing pioneer of modern medicine in ancient Greece, Hippocrates. Doctors have always recognized that there are several stages in the course of a severe burn case—if the patient lives. First is the period of immediate shock, the searing pain that sometimes passes all belief, all human endurance, the typical picture of the severely burned patient so familiar to all interns during their tour of duty in the emergency room.

This initial shock is not often very deep, usually it can be relieved by an injection of morphine and by pumping into the veins glucose or salt solution to boost a circulation temporarily depressed by the continual stream of nerve impulses pouring into the body from a burned area. Dr. Alfred Blalock, famed shock investigator, labeled it "neurogenic shock" years ago. Certainly this stage is different from the profound shock that develops later, although they may actually be only different phases in the development of the same picture.

The second period in burn shock begins very soon afterward, within the first twenty-four hours. It is the real danger period in severe cases. For a long time doctors were not sure just what was happening to these patients, why they rapidly went downhill in spite of the tremendous quantities of fluids pumped heroically into flagging circulations, why the blood pressure got lower, the blood darker with oxygen-lack, until finally they died of what appeared to be profound toxemia.

A few things they did know, however. One was that there was a great weeping from the burned areas and a sticky exudate soon developed. The simplest theory to explain the profound change in the patient was to say that some substance was absorbed into the body from the burned skin, a strange toxin that rapidly poisoned the entire body.

Some investigators still believe that there is a poison formed in the burned skin, and articles appear in medical journals describing methods of treatment to combat it. The treatment first devised was standard for burns until comparatively modern times, the "tannic acid" treatment. Certainly it did much to lower the mortality from burns when first introduced.

Briefly, tannic-acid treatment consisted of spraying the burned area with a solution of the acid, the same substance used to tan leather. A thick, leathery coagulation of the dead skin and the exudate that poured from it formed rapidly. The leathery coagulum effectively sealed off the burned area and stopped much of the weeping, certainly a helpful thing. This method was rapidly adopted by doctors everywhere and finally largely abandoned, but as recently as the beginning of our participation in World War II tannic acid was still listed as the treatment of choice in war burns.

Not everyone used it, however. Some surgeons used various dyes that seemed to accomplish the same thing. Others, when the sulfonamide drugs first became popular, used various solutions containing these new agents. But they all had one essential feature: production of a leathery coagulum over the burned area.

The very fact that medical scientists didn't stop with that accomplishment is evidence that they recognized tannic acid was not the ideal treatment. A lot of things were wrong with it. The main trouble was that all too frequently infection developed under the coagulum and pools of pus formed there, causing high-fever, toxemia, and depleting the reserve strength of a patient already skating on the thin edge. Another disadvantage was that widespread scarring occurred as the wounds slowly healed under the thick, leathery layer.

Still another set of researchers, in fact many sets, were tackling the problem from another angle. They weren't satisfied with the assumption that their patients died from a poison absorbed from burned tissues. They were investigating another problem at the same time, the problem of surgical shock, and were finding that the essential thing about shock was a sharp loss of blood plasma from the circulating blood.

They weren't sure just where the plasma went. There were a lot of theories, but the best one seemed to be that shock in some way injured the walls of the tiny capillary blood vessels all over the body and allowed the protein-containing plasma to seep through. The results were first a thickening of the blood called hemoconcentration, and then an inability of the circulation to maintain itself sufficiently so that the blood got plenty of oxygen, resulting in oxygen-lack with cyanosis. This picture of thick, dark blood was frequent in surgical shock, they realized, and they labeled it "oligemia," which means not enough blood.

But the blood looked like that in many burn cases, too! Given a patient with a severe burn treated early with morphine and fluid to relieve the pain and immediate shock, and treated with the then accepted tannic-acid method, there was often a picture of thick, dark blood, a failing circulation with falling blood pressure, delirium, and fear of impending disaster. Maybe the pictures were the same thing; it was a logical thought.

So laboratory workers got busy everywhere and started testing the blood of burned patients by putting it through the hematocrit test, whirling it in a centrifuge and separating the cells from the plasma. They tested the rate it fell through that ingenious little instrument for determining blood specific gravity, the falling-drop apparatus, and did actual chemical estimations of the blood proteins, with long banks of slender-necked Kjeldahl flasks sending pungent vapors into the hoods of the chemical laboratories.

They discovered an exciting thing, too. It was shock that occurred in severe burns. Actually it was easier to explain how shock took place in burns than in other cases, for they could see the plasma weeping from the burned areas, while in surgical shock they had to blame it on a mysterious loss into the tissues that no one entirely understands, even yet.

Articles appeared everywhere in the medical journals, advocating the use of blood transfusion, pectin solutions, acacia solutions, anything to replace the lost blood plasma. Remember, this was before a practical method of separating blood cells from plasma had been devised, a development largely brought about by World War II. When that arrived, the answer was simple; doctors poured plasma into burned patients, plasma and blood, too, for they knew that there was a sharp tendency toward anemia developing at about this time.

The mortality rate from burns took a sharp drop as soon as adequate plasma replacement began to be the accepted method of treatment, and it has been dropping ever since. Now a new compound called Dextran offers considerable hope of serving as a substitute for plasma, which is not always easy to obtain. Its molecule is large and does not easily pass through capillary walls. Dextran plus blood is extremely effective as a shock-alleviating agent.

Equally dramatic in some cases is the effect of the newest of the wonder drugs, ACTH and cortisone, often serving to keep desperately shocked patients alive until other therapy can pick up the slack.

Even though doctors now got their patients through the second period of plasma loss with these new methods of treatment, they still had a headache, for it was during this period of general toxemia that they often lost the fight that seemed already won. Almost all these burn cases became infected; pus developed under the eschars, the leathery tannings. The patients quickly showed the general picture of a severe infection, with fever, increased white blood counts, sometimes rapidly developing anemia, sometimes septicemia— and all too often, death. All kinds of dressings were tried, and anyone who sustained a severe burn years ago must still remember with a shudder the painful daily dressings, the hot compresses, and the salt baths.

Doctors were fighting heroically, meanwhile, to stem the effects of those violet-staining streptococci they found in the pus, but it was a long, slow fight. In fact, this stage merged into the next one in the burn picture, the stage of healing, and that was the most prolonged of all. Great scars formed, even in spite of thousands of skin grafts spotted about on the raw surface; joints were constricted by scars; features were drawn out of shape and required long series of plastic operations.

So, always searching for the perfect answer to the problem, medical researchers all over the world started hunting for the answer to the problem of infection in burns. A German chemist had the answer even then, but it was too unbelievable for anyone to realize yet, and so the parent of the sulfonamides, sulfanilamide, remained just a laboratory curiosity for years when it might have been saving thousands of lives.

Some surgeons took burn cases and put them into the operating rooms, gave them an anesthetic, cut away burned skin and tissue—in the operation French surgeons call *débridement*—and scrubbed the wounds clean with soap and water just as they scrubbed their hands before an operation. Then they covered them with a tannic-acid covering.

A few, however, used only a dressing with pressure. And they got results; there was no denying that. A patient who had his burned area treated as we now treat wounds, by removing damaged tissue, had less infection and less trouble afterward. The trouble was that in the case of a dangerously shocked patient they couldn't do all these things. In fact, it was all anyone could do to keep the patient alive, and the added burden of an anesthetic and a long surgical operation was often out of the question.

That pretty well stymied surgical treatment of large burns, but at about that time the sulfonamides appeared to aid in solving the problem. Doctors had been pouring these drugs into wounds and into abdominal cavities. Now they devised ingenious methods to put them in contact with the infected burned skin. The best method seemed to be one developed by Dr. Kenneth L. Pickrell, of Johns Hopkins, a preparation of sulfadiazine that formed a thin, transparent, flexible membrane over the burned areas. Thus the healing could take place under direct observation of the doctor through the dressing. It was ingenious and very satisfactory, but it still took an awful lot of time.

Meanwhile, a great disaster was in the making; America was rapidly approaching a war. Military surgeons were hunting for a practical, simple treatment for burns. The National Research Council, through its Division of Medical Sciences and its Committee on Surgery, composed of many of the country's leading surgeons, was also searching for a satisfactory treatment for burns. All the leading medical schools, too, were joining in this search.

At Harvard Medical School and the Massachusetts General Hospital, two research projects had been undertaken under stimulus of the Committee on Surgery of the National Research Council. One dealt with infections in burns and other wounds. Another dealt with disturbances inside the body that resulted from burns, the physiological side of the problem.

On the infection side, results were not long in developing. The question of local treatment of burns with the sulfonamide drugs was still being very widely discussed throughout the country. The value of these drugs in treating a large number of battle casualties had now apparently been adequately demonstrated at Pearl Harbor. Its power to prevent sepsis in wounds was unquestioned, but was it necessary to apply it locally in burns? Everybody recognized the danger, that you could not always tell how much of the drug would be absorbed into the body and could not always control the effective level. Did it work equally well when taken internally, where you could always exactly control the amount?

These questions were not long in being answered. Burn patients were given sulfonamide drugs and the blood concentration checked. Then fluid was taken from their burn blisters, the place where infection had always developed before these drugs came along. That, too, was tested for the concentration of the new drug. Results were gratifying, for the concentration in the blood and in the burn-blister fluid was approximately the same. This meant that when the drug was given by mouth or into the veins, it went directly to the spot where the battle against infection was being waged, the burned skin.

The question of whether to use the sulfonamides locally or generally or both was settled pretty effectively then. The local use was abandoned by many doctors treating burns. Later, of course, penicillin and the other antibiotics replaced sulfa drugs in treatment of burns and decided the question once and for all.

But it wasn't enough to know how to prevent infection from spreading, from raging through the body. What about keeping it from ever getting there in the first place? Researchers were studying that all over the country, too, just as they were at Harvard. And they were discovering an interesting thing. For a short time after the burn occurs, no bacteria can be grown from the burned skin. It is to all intents and purposes a sterile wound.

That finding knocked into a cocked hat the idea that burned skin was always infected skin. But where did the infection come from? It had to be from somewhere, that was certain. So again researchers began to look for the portal of entry. These things sound simple now, but they weren't then. First bacteriologists cultured the pus from infected burns. One set of germs they found were constantly present, and pretty malignant devils they were, too—the streptococci. Where did those "streps" come from, if they weren't there in the beginning?

Strangely enough the answer to that question had been given a full hundred years before by a half-crazy obstetrician in Vienna, named Semmelweis. In 1847 he showed how infection was carried by doctors who didn't wash their hands. But modern doctors, nurses, ward attendants, always wash their hands when treating burn cases. In fact, modern hospitals would not tolerate any such possibility of transmitting infection; instruments were used in changing those burn dressings and applying the moist compresses. The burned surface was not touched by hands at all, but the streps got there just the same, so there must be a reservoir of these troublemakers somewhere.

Well, there was, right in the throat of every patient in a ward, every doctor, every nurse, and every attendant. Each time someone coughs or sneezes, thousands or even millions of streptococci are sprayed out into the air. They hang there awhile, float around a little, then settle down into the dust and are periodically given a free ride through the air again when someone industriously sweeps the ward. Burn patients were treated routinely under great open cradles. What more simple way for the streptococci to get there than through the air, by means of the frequent dressings done in the morning routine just after the ward was swept and filled with dust-riding streps?

So a new routine was developed for handling burned cases. No *débridement* first, for study had shown that the burned skin was not infected. Simply cover the wounds immediately with sterile towels until they could be dressed correctly to prevent streptococci from getting to them. Then treat each burn just as if it were a surgical operation. Other investigators had proved that treating a burn this way cut down the incidence of infection, but they hadn't figured a way to prevent reinfection from dressing.

The original dressing for the burn was simple. Doctors, nurses, and assistants scrubbed up as for an operation, used sterile instruments and all ordinary precautions. When they took off the sterile towels they sometimes had to remove oil and grease slapped on the burn by some zealous but misguided amateur in first aid. But here again science was coming to the aid of medicine in discovering those odd chemicals now used in every household, the detergents. Then they covered the whole area with strips of fine-mesh vaselined gauze, sometimes impregnated with boric acid. Over this they put gauze dressings and over them soft pads of cotton and mechanics waste. Next they applied even compression, putting pressure everywhere but being careful not to constrict an arm or a leg or a toe or finger.

With this treatment, doctors even covered face burns, too, leaving only a couple of small holes for breathing and taking fluids. Pressure, they knew, tended to prevent weeping from the wound. The wounds were clean, so there was no need to change the dressing for five or ten days, particularly when the patient was taking drugs that prevented any further infection. And even when they were changed, the same procedure was repeated exactly so that no streps could get to this fresh, raw, burned flesh. What a departure from the old painful daily dressings that brought so much suffering to the patient, while effectively inoculating his burn with bacteria!

Other investigators hadn't been idle, either. They had already proved that blood plasma is the thing for burns, but they continued to study the whole problem of fluid replacement in those cases. Finally they worked out a scheme for keeping the blood at its normal levels in all the vital requirements, thus combating the early period of shock and the later period of anemia, toxemia, and general debilitation.

Doctors had known for a long time that it was better to cover raw, granulating surfaces with skin to prevent scarring, contractures, and hideous deformities, a tremendous psychological handicap to the unfortunate burn sufferer, sometimes so warping his thinking that he is no longer normal. But they knew also that it was a matter of weeks before their grafts would take, weeks while they soaked off the tannic-acid coagula, treated the raw surface with compresses and antiseptics to get rid of infections, and built up the rich pink covering that is called "granulation tissue." This was necessary for successful growing of the tiny skin islands then in use, called "small deep grafts," or sometimes just "pinch grafts."

A number of plastic surgeons hadn't been satisfied with this approach. They knew that, generally speaking, the best dressing for any raw surface is skin, the patient's own skin preferably. Skin from donors, even those with the same blood grouping, rarely takes permanently, although it is very often of tremendous temporary value.

Ingenious instruments were devised to shave a very thin layer of skin, most notable of which was the Padgett "dermatome," consisting of a metal drum that is rolled over previously prepared skin while a knife cuts an exactly predetermined thickness of skin from the patient's own body surface, leaving this paper-thin layer on the drum. Unlike the temperamental little pinch grafts, this new tissue-paper-thin layer would grow almost anywhere and large areas could be covered with it in only a short time—maybe ten or fifteen days —after the burn, cutting the entire recovery period from months to weeks and days.

No wonder few could really believe that the treatment of burns had been made so simple. Ideas like these usually take years to permeate into general knowledge, and undoubtedly would have in this case but for a great disaster that was at the same time a great blessing. For there occurred one of those strange machinations of fate, a disaster preparing against greater disasters.

On Saturday evening, November 28, 1942, the Cocoanut Grove, a night club in Boston, became a flaming holocaust of death and disaster. Fire raced through flimsy draperies while a crazed mass of people fought to escape. One hundred and fourteen casualties were brought to the Massachusetts General Hospital within a period of two hours, probably the greatest single flow of burned patients into any civilian hospital before Hiroshima and Nagasaki.

Fortunately the hospital staff were doubly prepared. Not only had catastrophe preparations been made under civilian-defense procedures—a blood bank had been established and plenty of blood and plasma were available—but research projects in the new treatments just described had been carried out here.

The result is history. What happened was described widely in newspapers and magazines, over the radio, by every route of communication, until there was no excuse for anyone not knowing that a new treatment of burns had been developed. Never before had such success been attained in healing burns. It was the final, incontrovertible proof that burns could be treated successfully on simple lines, by relieving shock, preventing infection, and grafting skin early to prevent scarring.

The system of treatment first used for victims of the Cocoanut Grove disaster has been widely adopted all over the world. A few modifications were inevitable and only added to its effectiveness. The sulfonamide drugs, lifesavers in preventing infections in burns, are definitely dangerous because of the decreased kidney function in burn cases, so penicillin and the various other antibiotic drugs were welcome improvements in the treatment.

Widely used in World War II and in Korea, the "bundling method" has proved its value. Research continues, of course, for a problem as grave as the burn threat in the Atomic Age is never really solved. Dextran and other agents that hold fluid inside the blood vessels; new methods of forming a sealing layer over burned areas, such as the use of aluminum powder; the shock-counteracting effect of ACTH and cortisone in the early stages—all are products of the marriage of science and surgery for the benefit of mankind. And in the great medical research centers of the country, skilled plastic surgeons are busy working their miracles of repair and reconstruction on those injured by burns and other agents.

20.

NEW FACES

─────────────────────────────────

Facial and jaw injuries—New strides in plastic surgery—Wiring of bone fragments—New noses from ribs—Use of diced cartilage—Molds from tantalum—New jaws from shinbones—New lips from scalp tissue—Removal of scars—Skin grafting—Elimination of stitches—Thromboplastics in affixing new skin—Whole-skin grafts from leg or abdomen—Replacement of muscles—New skin over jaws, new gums—Artificial replacements—Control of fingers on artificial hands

Plastic surgery, no matter how skilled the operator, cannot accomplish a miracle. Tissues that are lacerated, crushed, or burned heal only by the formation of fibrous tissue as scars. A surgeon cannot prevent those scars entirely, but he can, by applying the principles of plastic surgery developed in the past several decades, definitely keep these scars at a minimum, and place them where the natural creases and stress lines of the skin tend to minimize them almost to complete obscurity. He can remove unsightly scars and restore the normal contours of exposed portions of the body, like the face; that is near enough to a miracle to satisfy most victims.

Warfare accidents and civil-life disasters inevitably cause some injuries involving the face and jaws. In World War I there were many injuries to these structures. The impetus this gave the baby science of plastic and maxillofacial surgery resulted in such advances as split-skin grafts, the Padgett dermatome, the acrylic dental splint, facial moulage for the planning of plastic repair, external methods of fixation of fractured jaws, and a succession of discoveries too long to mention.

Trench warfare in World War I resulted in a disproportionately large number of injuries to the head and face. Early in the conflict it was recognized that specially trained personnel were needed to handle these injuries, if the least deformity was to result. So surgeon-dentist teams were formed in the various theaters to advise and direct the treatment of wounds involving the face and jaws.

In World War II and in the Korean conflict, surgeons and dentists were trained in the principles of treating injuries to the face and jaws. Almost every front-line hospital, and certainly the evacuation hospitals where the first definitive treatment was usually given, had available surgeons familiar with this field of surgery, ably assisted by dentists skilled in treating such injuries.

Some things about face and jaw wounds—involving either the lower jaw, the mandible, or the upper, the maxilla—must always be considered. The blood supply to the structures of the face is unusually great, greater than that of any other portion of the body. This means that face wounds tend to heal well and without infection. Rarely is it necessary to cut away much tissue in this region; usually it is inadvisable. Certainly, wound excision, advised for wounds elsewhere in the body to prevent gas gangrene, is unnecessary and not desirable, since structures such as pieces of bone and skin and sections of the intricate system of muscles controlling facial expression may be removed when they could serve much better if left in place. The large blood supply also means that face and jaw injuries are subject to free hemorrhage; unless proper first aid is administered early, the victims may die from loss of blood.

The upper jaw contains air cells, called sinuses, whose walls are rather thin and therefore are crushed easily. Failure to restore the walls of these sinuses as nearly as possible to their former state will result in depression and deformity of the cheeks. The same is true of the nose. Failure to adjust the maxillary bones of the upper jaw to their normal positions will considerably alter the appearance of the mouth. In the lower jaw, loss of sections of bone will destroy the mobility of the jaw. What is worse, with the loss of any large portion of the lower jaw, the attachments of the tongue are released and it tends to fall backward into the throat. Suffocation from respiratory-passage obstruction by the tongue during transportation is a very present danger and must always be considered.

Realizing that the initial care these casualties receive may affect seriously their future welfare, the American Army very early made provisions to train medical personnel in the care of face and jaw injuries. After reviewing the cases occurring in World War I, pioneer plastic surgeon Dr. Vilray P. Blair concluded that proper early care not only was lifesaving but preserved tissue that could not be replaced later, prepared the casualty for early evacuation, and reduced greatly the reconstructive surgery later necessary to restore the facio-maxillary casualty to normal civil life.

With modern methods of plastic repair and facial reconstruction, coupled with the miraculous things done with prosthetic appliances, there is little reason why any facio-maxillary casualty should not eventually face the world with the knowledge that, though scarred, he is certainly no object of loathing.

With the popularity of the automobile, which afforded an excellent means whereby more people were able to destroy themselves, more or less completely, between the two world wars than have been destroyed in any war, plastic surgeons and reconstructive specialists had a great mass of material on which to work. In general, automobile-accident cases were brought to the hospitals earlier, resulting in far less infection and far less interruption of the planned course of repair because of infection.

Military casualties, unfortunately, could not usually be evacuated so quickly, although air transport, particularly during the Korean conflict, did much to speed the facio-maxillary casualty to the trained plastic surgeon in a fixed base hospital. Possibilities for infection were, therefore, greater in military cases. Fortunately, however, the widespread use of penicillin and sulfonamide drugs gave surgeons a mighty weapon in fighting infection.

With the beginning of World War II, training nuclei were established in many centers over the country—in Philadelphia

Rochester, and at crack Army Walter Reed General Hospital, to name but three. From these were preached the doctrines that did so much to further the efficient handling of these injuries and prevent the deformities that inevitably follow incorrect application of the simple basic principles of facio-maxillary surgery.

The person who first reaches such a casualty, whether on the battlefield or by the roadside, can do much. He must control hemorrhage immediately, with pressure dressings applied so as to support the injured tissues without increasing the injury. Second, he can maintain a proper airway so the patient will not suffocate from the pressure of his own swollen tongue against the back of his throat. If necessary the person giving first aid may grasp the tongue and draw it forward, clearing the respiratory passage. The casualty is then hurried back to the hospital by litter—face down.

The importance of placing the face down, which promotes the exit of mucus and blood from the respiratory passages and prevents the tongue from dropping back against the roof of the mouth and causing suffocation, cannot be too heavily stressed.

At the hospital, hemorrhage is controlled by locating each bleeding vessel and tying it off. The wound is cleansed carefully and any foreign matter removed, for even the great blood supply of the facial structures cannot prevent infection around dirty foreign material, such as clothing. War surgeons were careful not to remove from the facio-maxillary wounds any fragments of bone that had attachments to other tissues. Upon the viability of a small piece of bone may depend the final continuity of the jaw; leaving it in place may preclude the later necessity of several bone grafts.

Fractures and bits of bone must be restored to approximately their normal positions and held there by pressure, often by fixing the upper and lower jaws together by means of wire loops drawn together by rubber bands. Should anything interfere with the patient's breathing, the rubbers can be cut quickly and the mouth opened widely to permit traction on the tongue. Surgeons are careful to put skin and mucous membrane flaps back into as near their original positions as possible, but they avoid the mistake of tightly sewing up wounds of the floor of the mouth.

Since the mouth cavity is teeming with bacteria, tightly suturing a wound of the floor of the mouth may bottle up infection beneath it, allowing the inflammation to spread backward in the tissue spaces of the neck, or descend along the fascia planes down into the chest, to cause frequently fatal inflammation of the vital structures of the mediastinum there. Where infection seems likely, surgeons make incisions for drainage, and with this they give large doses of the antibiotic drugs as a formidable armor against infection.

Plastic surgeons insist on a meticulous repair of skin lacerations, shifting sections of upper or lower jaw, which may still not be entirely in position, into the optimum location for healing back to their normal contours. Fractured jaws are treated and the fragments held in their normal relationships by wiring, or by one of the transparent plastic splints molded exactly to fit the tooth pattern of the individual and then wired immovably into place.

The art of replacing bone defects about the face and jaw structures has been brought to a high degree of perfection. Several methods are used, each specially suited for a particular deformity. Loss of a section of the nose can be corrected by removing from the front end of one of the ribs a section of the white gristle, or cartilage, that forms an elastic connection between the actual rib and the sternum, or breastbone. This cartilage is soft and can be shaped and whittled to fit the contours of the feature to be replaced. Through incisions placed inside the mouth or the nose, where no scars will result, strips of cartilage can be moved into place and anchored, forming a supporting framework over which the skin can be repaired or grafted, restoring the normal contours of the face.

For filling large defects an ingenious method of cartilage graft can be used. Here the cartilage is removed from the rib ends and diced up into hundreds of tiny fragments. These are then sewn just beneath the skin in the area to be repaired and the tissues held in the position in which they are to heal by means of a latex rubber mold. The bits of cartilage then heal together into a firm fibrous layer, leaving a strong support to restore the original outlines of the face in the area where the defect occurred.

Still another and equally ingenious replacement is carried out by molding a shell of the new miracle metal, tantalum. The possibilities of this metal seem endless; dentists envision the time when artificial teeth may be screwed directly into the bone or whole sets wired into place immovably without disturbing the normal life processes of the jaws.

Where sections of the lower jaw are gone completely, they, too, can be replaced by bone or cartilage graft. One type of bone graft shaves thin layers from the shin and transfers them to the bone defect in the lower jaw, where they set up new growth processes and shortly bridge the defect with strong healthy bone. Another uses a section of rib. Dental prosthetists can mold artificial dentures that support the teeth and also tissues that may have lost their bony framework. Almost the entire upper or lower jaw can be replaced by these prosthetic appliances, supporting the lips and cheek and giving the face once more its normal contour.

In the matter of replacing skin defects, plastic surgeons have proved equally ingenious. A lost upper lip can be supplied by elevating a strip of scalp above the hairline, grafting a thin film of skin on the under surface to act as a new mucous membrane for the lip, then swinging the whole thing down across the nose and into place to form an upper lip, complete with mustache, if desired. Scars that distort normal appearance can be removed and the skin edges brought together with tiny needles and fine thread, if the skin is loose enough to allow the edges to heal without tension. Tension results in scars, so no tension must occur in plastic-surgery wounds.

Skin grafts to cover areas from which scars have been removed can be of several types. One method of cutting grafts has proved so satisfactory that it has largely supplanted other types of graft for most plastic skin grafting. No longer are the multiple transplants called pinch grafts used to any great extent. They cover large burned areas very effectively, it is true, but the final appearance of the skin is unsightly, and of course they have no part about the face.

The new "split thickness" grafts contain only a part of the

total thickness of the skin, leaving the donor site free to heal without any scarring. The dermatome, devised by ingenious plastic surgeon Earl C. Padgett, is an amazingly efficient machine for cutting grafts of any desired thickness.

But here, too, science has discovered something new. Formerly it was necessary to attach the skin grafts carefully with hundreds of tiny stitches and then to maintain a firm pressure dressing lest secretions from the raw surface of the wound accumulate beneath the graft and prevent its "taking" on the grafted area. Then some workers, notably Dr. M. E. Sano, of Philadelphia, demonstrated that blood plasma could be clotted by the addition of certain clot-forming substances also present in the blood.

Briefly, the method consists of breaking up the white blood cells to release this "thromboplastic" substance, which is then mixed with blood plasma and painted on the sheet of skin cut by the dermatome. A firm adhesive clot forms rapidly between the skin graft and the area to be grafted, no dressings are necessary, and the growth of tiny blood vessels into the skin from the surrounding areas takes place much more rapidly than in a graft held in place by sutures in the ordinary way.

In the face, however, it is usually desirable to have grafts that contain the whole thickness of the skin. Here plastic surgeons ingeniously use what are called "pedicle flaps." These are tubes of skin, raised up on the leg, arm, shoulder, or even abdomen, neck, or scalp. A week or so later one end is detached and restitched into place higher up, sometimes on an arm. As soon as a firm healing has taken place between the ends of the tube and its new attachment, and new blood vessels have grown into this end of the skin tube, the lower end is detached. In this way it is quite possible to carry a tube of skin, cartwheel fashion, up the body and into place on the face. Or even more ingeniously, it can be carried to an arm, then the arm is raised and fixed beside the face, to which the graft is then transferred to fill the defect. There is no end to the uses that can be made of these pedicled flaps by dexterous plastic surgeons.

So fine are the wound lines from delicate plastic procedure that they are often not visible except at close range. Where muscles are lost, they can be supplied by shifting sections of other facial muscles.

An ingenious method of using strips of living fascia, the tough, fibrous tissue that covers the muscles of the leg and other parts of the body, or tantalum wire, can maintain the normal contour of the mouth and eyelids by slinging them from the cheek bone, the whole being accomplished beneath the skin where it will not show. Even scars can be hidden by a paste used to cover birthmarks that is hardly distinguishable from the surrounding skin when properly applied.

Where the lower jaw, lip, and skin over the chin region have been lost, the problem becomes more difficult and the attack more gradual. First, a tube of skin must be developed on the chest, the neck, or elsewhere. The surgeon next cuts a thin graft with the dermatome or some similar instrument, wraps it around a mold of dental compound, and then slips this inside the original skin tube, thus obtaining a completely lined tube, with both inside and outside covered by skin.

Thus three aims are accomplished before the jaw region itself is approached. The inner lining of the new tube graft serves as a compartment into which the new cartilage or bone graft is slipped to replace the lost section of lower jawbone. And when the outer layer of skin covering the tube is slit, there is left an outer covering of skin for the lip and an inner covering that takes the place of the membrane of the lip and gum.

With all this preliminary preparation made, the tissues remaining in the lower-jaw region can now be freed, lifted up, and a bed prepared into which the graft will fit. The graft, taken from rib, rib cartilage, or other bone, is properly attached in its new home. The jaw is completely reconstructed in this way, the attachments of the tongue put in their proper place, the grafted jaw splinted with an acrylic mold against the upper jaw to allow healing.

To see the before and after results of these detailed procedures, as they are carried out in the great surgical centers by the leading plastic experts of the country, leaves one filled with awe at what the hand of man, bulwarked by science, can do to remodel the damaged human body.

In some cases, it must be realized, loss of tissue is so great that rather than try to replace the normal contours by many plastic operations, a prosthetic appliance must be molded to replace the lost section of the face. This is particularly true of older people and the defects that result from the treatment of large superficial cancers. So marvelously made are these prostheses that they cannot be distinguished from the original organ by anyone who does not know that an artificial appliance is in place.

Basic step in this preparation of a prosthetic appliance is making a mold of the area. Here comes in the use of moulage. Moulage means literally "mold." For making the original molds, a hydrocolloidal substance is frequently used. The hydrocolloid melts at a low temperature and can be brushed on the face of the subject until an even, smooth layer covers the features. In a few minutes it sets into a perfect cast of the part to be treated, and can then be removed. This shell, or negative, is used to make a positive model of the face.

Working on this model, it is possible to build up the facial contours to the desired outline, and from this the actual prosthesis can be made of latex or some other suitable substance. Colored to blend in with the skin shade of the face, the prosthesis is put on and taken off like a pair of glasses, removing instantly the visible deformity. By means of these miraculous face savers, many a person today is able to walk the streets unnoticed, despite the loss of a nose or an entire section of the jaw.

Perhaps the most fascinating of all plastic procedures is the cineplastic amputation. While an ordinary artificial arm does have many uses, doctors have long sought for a means of controlling the fingers of such a hand to permit more use. The answer—or the beginnings of an answer, for the whole thing is still in what might be termed the experimental stage —has indicated that the results may be very good indeed.

Briefly, the cineplastic operation aims to create connections between the remaining arm muscles and the artificial fingers corresponding to those they controlled before amputation. For a long time this posed a problem, for it was impossible to attach living tendons to mechanical fingers without inevitable infection. This new operation leaves no open wounds and thereby obviates the difficulty.

On the surface of the skin several inches back of the amputation stump, the plastic surgeon makes a skin flap over the group of muscles controlling flexion of the fingers. He lifts up this flap, leaving one end attached, and sews the edges together to form a tube, perhaps an inch and a half long. Then through the muscles beneath the skin tube he makes a tunnel, through which he pulls the tube. When it comes out on the other side, he sews the edges of the tube to the edge of the skin from which it was cut away in the first place. Thus there is formed a skin-lined tube going entirely through the muscle, very much as if you were to thrust a heavy needle through the arm. The exposed muscle is now covered with a small skin graft and the tube allowed to heal in place.

When healing is complete, there is a tube of skin completely through the muscle, and into it is inserted a wooden or metal peg. When the muscle contracts, the skin tube and the peg are thus moved back and forth along the arm. The whole operation is then repeated on the other side of the arm, this time tunneling the extensor group of muscles, which control the extension of the fingers, and a peg is again inserted through this tube of skin.

Now comes the amazing part. When a properly made artificial hand and arm is slipped over the stump, and the two pegs are connected, the flexor one to the flexor controls of the fingers, and the extensor one to the extensor controls, the patient can open and close his artificial fingers. Thus an effective hand is made with which the patient soon learns to do many things he did before amputation.

Plastic surgery, like many other specialties in medicine, was given a tremendous shot in the arm by war-time advances. With this start, future advances promise to push it to even greater heights of accomplishment in a field that can relieve one of the most acute forms of mental torture—the shame of "being different."

21.

PSYCHOLOGY FOR SURGEONS

Emotions and their influence on disease—Autonomic nervous system again—Digestive tract especially susceptible—Ulcers—Nervous colitis—When psychiatry supplants surgery

Psychologists say, "The abdomen is the sounding board for the emotions." Forward-looking surgeons agree that if more of their brothers of the scalpel-wielding clan kept this in mind, there would be fewer unnecessary operations. Certainly hardly a day passes in the office of the successful surgeon when he does not see at least one person, usually a woman, who has been turned into a "surgical cripple" because the influence of the emotions on body functions was not recognized early enough.

So conscious have the great teaching centers become of the importance of considering the psychology of patients—even those presenting themselves for such ordinary surgical conditions as an attack of acute appendicitis—that staff psychologists and psychiatrists now work in close conjunction with the surgeons in evaluating all candidates for surgery. All this, of course, is just another phase of the fascinating new science of emotions and their influence on disease called psychosomatic medicine.

A great surgeon has laid down a dictum for students that the true measure of a surgeon's ability is not in knowing when to operate but in knowing when not to operate. To withhold the scalpel when the patient comes prepared and expecting, perhaps insisting on operation, requires moral and financial courage. To the credit of the science of surgery, more and more surgeons are practicing this kind of courage, recognizing the importance of psychosomatic medicine, and are setting out to learn something about this influence on the body exerted by the mental processes—in short, more surgeons are recognizing the importance of psychology in their profession.

Let us recapitulate quickly some facts from an earlier chapter. The interdependence of emotions and body functions comes about through a very specialized portion of the nervous system called the autonomic, or more popularly but less correctly the sympathetic nervous system.

Thought processes are carried out, of course, by the brain in the cerebral lobes. Here the function of will decides what will be done and initiates messages that tell the muscles or other organs what to do. Some functions of the body, however, require much more freedom of action. These are the functions vital to carrying on the ordinary life-preserving processes of respiration, digestion, circulation, and the function of the glands. To control these activities, the body uses a nearly autonomous nervous system called the autonomic. This automatic nervous system consists of a chain of small nodes of nerve cells located beside the spine and connected, by slender roots called rami, with the spinal cord and the central or voluntary portion of the nervous system. From these ganglia, a network of tiny nerves goes out to all the organs, controlling their function.

But specialization occurs even within the autonomic nervous system. Actually there are two departments, maintaining a constant system of checks and balances on each other. Take for example, the arteries carrying blood throughout the body. Distributed to all arteries are sets of nerve fibers from two sections of the autonomic system, the sympathetic and the parasympathetic divisions. One set, the sympathetic, tends to cause arteries to constrict and grow smaller, decreasing blood flow; the other, the parasympathetic, causes dilatation or increase in the size of an artery augmenting the blood current. The amount of blood flowing through an artery at any given time depends on the balance between these two influences.

An example of how this set of checks and balances works occurs three times a day when food is eaten. The thrice-daily stoking of the digestive tract with a large quantity of food sets it into a period of intensive activity. For the digested food to be absorbed properly into the body, a marked increase in the blood supply to the small intestine is necessary. This is accomplished first by an overbalance in favor of blood-vessel dilatation in the intestinal arteries and, to compensate for this, an overbalance in favor of constriction in the rest of the arteries. As a result the blood supply to the brain is cut down, mental functions are poorly carried out, and we become sleepy and listless. The body uses perfect sense when it suggests an afternoon nap just after a heavy midday meal.

Thus can be seen how the body, without conscious thought, takes care of these vital functions. But the central nervous system does maintain a close check on the functions of the autonomic. For instance, when the breath is held, carbon dioxide accumulates in the blood as a waste product of body function. This increase in carbon-dioxide concentration affects a very specialized little group of cells in the lower part of the brain called the respiratory center, which in turn acts through the autonomic nerve trunks and the muscles of respiration to cause an overpowering impulse to breathe.

In the same way the rate of breathing is slowed or increased, depending on the concentration of carbon dioxide in the blood to the cells of the respiratory center. Other centers control blood pressure and similar vital functions.

A classic example of the body's constant fight to maintain a normal situation is in shock. Shock, as already pointed out, results from a loss of the fluid portion of the blood, causing increased viscosity and a decrease in the total blood volume. With less blood to pump, the heart has to work faster and the pulse rate goes up, due to autonomic control. In addition, the smaller blood vessels contract everywhere to try to make the volume of the circulation conform with the volume of blood available to circulate through it. As long as these compensations by the autonomic nervous system continue to function, blood pressure is maintained and the circulation keeps up. When they are no longer able to compensate, the circulation fails, the brain does not get enough oxygen, unconsciousness and death ensue.

Examples could be given endlessly of automatic functions—

the speed-up of the muscular contractions of the intestinal wall when there is food in the stomach; the stimulation of the adrenal glands by the emotion of fear, leading to a tremendous outpouring of adrenalin; the spasm of the esophagus and upper end of the stomach that gives you a lump in your throat; the tingle that goes down your spine when you listen to the *Star-Spangled Banner*. All these are automatic functions carried out by the autonomic nervous system without orders from the brain.

If the automatic nervous system were just that, completely automatic, people would undoubtedly live longer and much saner lives. But it is not. Any disturbance of thought processes, particularly emotional experiences, turmoil, conflict, or strain, are reflected immediately in the function of the autonomics and may seriously affect vital functions of the body. It is to this unfortunate violence of emotional effect that psychologists refer when they say, "The abdomen is the sounding board of the emotions."

Were the effects limited to the abdomen, we would all be better off, but again they are not. Emotional explosions affect every part of the body and interfere with all functions. To the extent that the resistance of the autonomic nervous system is low to emotional "spillovers," we are victims of that commonest of all nervous afflictions, what the psychologists call "psychoneurosis" or "increased psychomotor activity."

It is well established now that the digestive tract is peculiarly liable to be affected by the emotions. Excitement brings a lump to your throat, evidence that your emotional increase has spilled over into the autonomic nervous system and has set into spasm certain circular muscles of the esophagus and stomach called sphincters. If you are very sensitive, the reaction may continue to a point where sphincters remain in spasm and vomiting will result, a familiar enough reaction to many people when under nervous strain.

Less well understood is the process by which the development and healing of stomach and duodenal ulcers is affected by the emotions, yet every gastroenterologist will tell you that a continued disturbance of emotions absolutely insures against the healing of an ulcer, whatever the treatment, while subsidence of an emotional conflict brings about rapid healing with no other treatment.

Of special interest in this connection is the work, recently reported, in which the stomach-wall reactions to emotional stimuli were observed through an artificial opening into the stomach, made because a stricture of the esophagus prevented swallowing of food. The color of the stomach lining reflected exactly the emotional stimulus given the patient, indicating that in susceptible persons the local damage to the stomach wall from impeded blood supply by spasm may be largely instrumental in causing the ulcer.

Perhaps less well known to the public, but again a common symptom recognized by the doctor, is the effect of the emotions on the function of the colon. Nervous colitis, spastic colitis, even to a certain extent the much more severe and dangerous ulcerative colitis, are all largely conditioned by the influence of emotions on the functioning of the large bowel. The symptoms of discomfort, gassiness, belching, and distension, so often associated with so-called nervous indigestion, are all merely manifestations of the imbalance of the autonomic nervous system caused by emotional tension.

What, then, does all this have to do with surgery? Often a great deal. The emotional-sounding-board effects in the abdomen tend to display themselves as pain in the right side, usually low down and close to the region of the appendix. Just why this overstimulation of the autonomic nervous system with spasm of the muscles of the wall of the digestive and reproductive tracts, should result in right-sided abdominal pain any more than in pain anywhere else in the abdomen is still a mystery. But every surgeon knows that any generalized disturbance of the abdomen will cause right-sided pain at least twice as frequently as it causes pain elsewhere.

The public is appendix-conscious, and rightly so, for only by this appendix consciousness will patients present themselves early enough to prevent rupture and peritonitis in the real appendicitis case. So this right-sided pain brings the patient to the doctor complaining of appendicitis.

The family doctor sends the patient to the surgeon with the same diagnosis, and the surgeon is on the spot. He must either operate or refute the opinion of both the patient and the doctor, thereby probably losing both the patient and the business of the referring physician, who is miffed by this refutation of his diagnosis. Here is a case where to operate is simple, but not to operate requires a great deal of courage. Fortunately, most real surgeons have this courage; unfortunately, some so-called surgeons do not.

Let's take a common example. A patient—young, beautiful, expensively dressed, and wearing a mink jacket—consults the surgeon because of persistent attacks of pain in the right side of the abdomen. A diagnosis of chronic appendicitis has been made and in a few cases—a very few cases—may be correct. The unwary surgeon operates, finds nothing wrong with the appendix, but is gratified to see that the patient improves rather markedly in the first few weeks after operation. Then she returns with the same complaint. Very often she leaves the puzzled doctor and goes to another, who feels that her trouble now is from adhesions following the operation. Again he operates, finds adhesions of no significance, but is pleased with temporary improvement, only to have the patient return in a few weeks with the same complaint.

A third surgeon, consulted by the patient in her eternal hunt for relief, feels that the uterus is out of place and performs a suspension of the uterus. By this time the patient is almost a complete surgical and psychological cripple. It is doubtful if she can ever again be anything but a fretful invalid.

Now, in some way or another, she finds her way to a surgeon who appreciates the importance of psychological study in cases like this and refers her to a psychiatrist. Disgusted with surgery, she may consult a psychiatrist herself.

Psychological questioning soon brings out the fact that she is married to a man much older than herself, is not in love with her husband, and has developed an attachment for someone less well off financially but more attractive physically. The conflict between her love for the impecunious admirer and her love for the luxury given her by her husband, coupled with a lack of sexual attraction between them, has caused an emotional turmoil that has spilled over into the autonomic nervous system and so disturbed the gastrointestinal tract that the right-sided pain has resulted.

Each operation temporarily salved the recurrent emotional crises. The excitement of visits by friends, expensive presents from her husband, perhaps an opportunity to dazzle the impecunious lover with the legal display of charms allowed by dainty bed jackets, negligees, and gowns, all acted to soothe disturbed emotions. Three operations have done nothing to benefit this patient. What was needed all along was some sound psychiatric advice.

A much less spectacular, but more prevalent, psychosomatic problem confronted surgeons during the Korean conflict and World War II. Armed service medical officers in dispensaries treating servicemen's dependents called it "army-wife syndrome." Here the emotional stimulus was much simpler and less dramatic. Absence of husband, loss of the traditional security that is the right of the wife and mother, worry about whether the husband would come home, coupled with lowered income, perhaps loss of a maid, and in many cases the care of small children—all these worked together to give an emotional wallop that often broke down even the strongest barriers of will.

The same pain occurred, right-sided, worse after a day of looking after the house and the children and intensified by the withdrawal into herself with which many a woman tried to fight the loneliness for her absent husband. Nagged by persistent discomfort, the patient was certain that her appendix was involved, or that her reproductive organs were not functioning well. Confirming these suspicions in her own mind, a disturbance of the menstrual rhythm occurred, a symptom familiar to all gynecologists in patients suffering emotional strain. Cancer phobia may also occur, and a complicating train of symptoms simulating disease of almost any organ in the abdomen.

The patient consulted a doctor, satisfied that her trouble required operation. She was examined, and perhaps a small cyst was found in one ovary or a slight malposition of the uterus. Gynecologists examining hundreds of women have repeatedly found these conditions in normal people, with no symptoms and causing no trouble.

If the army wife was lucky, she found a doctor who was psychosomatic-conscious, who kept in mind the precipitating emotional factors obviously at work in her body. He may not have been able to do very much about her emotional problem, although he could refer her to agencies set up to do what they could to make the burden of the left-at-home wife less intolerable. But he could explain to her intelligently and quietly just what was happening and suggest outlets for her emotional tension that might act as "blow-off valves" and prevent some of the physical symptoms that distressed her. Most important, he could assure her that she did not need an operation.

Not always does this type of case reach an understanding surgeon; much more often the patient is advised to be operated on, the familiar statement being "to remove a cyst from the ovary and suspend the uterus, removing the appendix at the same time." Competent and conservative gynecological surgeons recognize that there are some cases in which such operations are necessary, notably in cases of sterility, but their number is very, very small. Many outstanding specialists in surgery of the reproductive system do not perform half a dozen such operations a year.

Even when an operation is to be performed, the emotional state of the patient markedly influences the final result. Almost every hospital can give records of patients who came into the hospital for an ordinary operation, a hernia or an appendix, with the profound conviction that they were going to die—and did, although the operation was uneventful. Time spent in applying sound psychological principles to quell the turbulent emotions of surgical patients is not wasted. Anesthetists learned long ago that their patients took a better anesthetic if they were given a good sleep the night before with a mild sedative, and came to the operating room with senses dulled by a hypodermic.

Cancer patients particularly need assurance and the calming effect of mild psychotherapy, often consisting of nothing more than a confidential chat with the surgeon about their chances of surviving the operation and obtaining a cure from it. Once these things are explained, patients rarely dread the operation or the anesthetic. The prospect of a cure eclipses in their quieted minds any apprehension they might have had of the outcome.

Already included in the postgraduate curriculum of several famous medical centers, psychology for surgeons is rapidly being recognized for what it is—an important weapon in the armamentarium of the operator, in many cases far more valuable even than the scalpel. With the strain of living under the shadow of the hydrogen bomb, it is very important for the surgeon who would be true to his calling to know when *not* to operate.

22.

SURGERY CURES CANCER

Cures by X-ray and radium—Potentialities of atom-splitting in creating new radioactive substances for cancer treatment—How cancers develop—Cancer of the breast—The lymphatic vessels and secondary cancer growths—Cancer of the prostate gland, treatment by operation and female hormones—Benign tumors—Where cancers grow—Heredity in cancer—Cancer of the skin, of the stomach, intestines, rectum, uterus, cervix, lung, pancreas—Surgery in these cases

The United States is growing older.

This fact is not quite so simple as it looks to casual observation. Modern public-health methods, the tremendous advances in medical science, the consistent efforts of the medical profession to put itself out of business by keeping people from growing ill and dying—all these have combined to make the average age of the population considerably greater than it was ten years ago. In short, we are rapidly becoming a world composed of a larger and larger percentage of older people.

But age carries with it certain liabilities, perhaps the greatest of which is the increased incidence of cancer. Already the second-ranking cause of all deaths, cancer would bid fair to increase its toll were it not for continuous progress in diagnosing and treating malignant disease in the early stages, when it is amenable to treatment.

Cancer can be cured by surgery. There is no real reason for the pessimism with which the general population regards a diagnosis of cancer. It is not the worst thing that can happen

227

to anyone; a few other diseases kill with much more certainty than cancer in even its more virulent forms. The solution to cancer, so far as present scientific research and knowledge will let us state, lies in two principles—early surgery and adequate surgery.

Some malignant tumors are cured by radiation, either X-ray or radium or both. The new methods of creating radioactive substances called isotopes in the atomic pile have already extended considerably the field of radiation therapy, particularly in the control of recurrent cancer. And continuing research in the hormone field promises much in controlling certain types of malignant disease, notably that of the breast and prostate gland. Certainly few surgeons will deny the value of supplemental radiation treatment in many types of cancer. But by and large the best way to get rid of cancer is to remove it with the scalpel, and most modern methods of treatment hinge on this approach.

Cancer has been surrounded by a lot of scientific mumbo-jumbo, created perhaps perfectly naturally in the efforts to explain something for which there seems no adequate explanation. Simply expressed, a cancer is a lawless growth of body cells. Let us take a simple parallel. A solid citizen lives for years in a community, taking his normal place, performing all the activities that are a part of being a good citizen. In short, he is a unit in the society in which he exists, fundamentally like every other unit. Then one day he runs amuck and starts damaging his fellow men and taking over property that isn't his. From that moment on he is branded as an outlaw, and society seeks to get rid of him unless he can be made a useful citizen once again by less stern measures.

Exactly this sequence of events occurs when a cancer develops. During the early growth of human beings, in the period when the embryo is developing in the womb of the mother, a very rapid growth of body cells takes place. This has to be, if the embryo is to reach its normal size and development by birth. This growth continues after birth, but at a considerably diminishing rate, until it stops altogether in later life.

When it begins to live, the embryo individual is only one cell, formed by the fusion of the male and female sex cells, the ovum and the spermatozoön. This newly formed cell begins to divide immediately and growth takes place. Very early in the division process, the body begins to develop very definite specialism in its cells. Some grow to be skin, some bone, some muscle—in short, all the tissues of the body. But this is lawful growth, the normal expanding of a family, each member of which bears a close resemblance to the others. This growth follows certain natural laws by which legs, for instance, normally grow to the same length.

Sometimes, even this early, a few cells get out of hand and a tumor that we call an embryoma results. These embryomas retain the characteristics of embryonic cells, they grow rapidly, but they no longer obey the laws. They grow all over the place, invading other organs, reaching vital centers, and shortly the individual is killed by the outlaw developing inside its own body.

In the same way, cancers develop later in life. Under some stimulus—more about that later—cells begin to grow unlawfully. Let us take for example the female breast, one of the more frequent locations for cancer. The breast glands normally perform the function of secreting milk. Every structure in the breast is subordinated to that function. The breasts increase markedly in size and in the number of functioning gland units with pregnancy. But this is lawful growth, and the cells resemble other breast cells.

Now let a few cells in the breast begin a lawless growth. They may look superficially like normal breast cells, but changes soon appear that tell the pathologist looking through his microscope that these are outlaw cells, changes in the size of the nuclei of the cells, the way the dark material in the center of the cell is arranged, the size and shape of the cells. The pathologist can also tell how bad the outlaws are from their appearance. The closer they resemble normal breast cells, the less dangerous they are as cancers. The more they resemble embryonic cells, just growing for the sake of growing, the more dangerous they are, the quicker they cause trouble. But the important thing is that in the beginning there is a single nest of these outlaw cells in the breast, usually appearing as a lump of varying size.

If no surgeon is available, or if the person with the lump

goes on trying to convince herself that the growth is nothing and she shouldn't worry about it, the second stage of this outlawry of cells begins. This is the stage of spread. The outlaws begin to "muscle in" on the normal activity of the community. They do this usually by several paths. First is direct extension, growing into the tissues surrounding them. In the early stages this is limited to the organ in which they began; then the invasion extends to surrounding organs.

A second route of expansion is along the channels that drain fluid from around the cells, the lymphatic vessels. There is a vast network of these vessels in the body, roughly paralleling the veins. But the difference is that all along these lymph channels are situated little substations, called lymph nodes, which pick up unwanted things riding through on the lymph stream.

Let us take an example of how these lymph nodes work. When you get a sore toe, streaks run up your leg and a lump forms in the groin. This means that the infection has spread from the original sore toe up the lymphatic channels toward the blood stream, the lump forming when the lymph node tries to filter out the infection and itself becomes infected.

Cancer works in the same way, spreading along the lymphatics and, when it reaches a lymph gland or node, developing a secondary cancer, an individual nest of outlaw cells. As the cancer grows an increasingly wider range of lymph nodes become involved, until finally each new outlaw nest may be as dangerous as the original one.

But cancer spreads in still another way, and this is usually the last to occur, by seeding, or metastasis. This means simply that in the process of growth the outlaw cells burst into small blood vessels, break off, and are carried away through the body. They then lodge in other regions and again set up new nests of outlaw cells. Strangely enough, they seem to prefer certain areas. For example, prostate cancers frequently metastasize—that's the name for this seeding process—in bones, especially the spine. Certain types of bone cancers go to the lungs.

Even when metastasis has occurred, however, the situation is not hopeless by any means. A dramatic example of this concerns cancer of the prostate, the gland located just outside the bladder in men, which often enlarges and interferes with the work of the kidneys and bladder.

Surgeons learned some time ago that prostatic cancer seems to be affected by sex hormones; in fact, it is generally known that many cancers, notably the breast in females, are so affected. So they tried the effects of removing the sex glands in patients who apparently had hopeless cancers of the prostate with metastasis to bones.

The results were startling. The sharp reduction in male sex hormone following operation often caused the bone metastasis to disappear, and the original growth in the prostate shrank remarkably. Some cancer surgeons carried this idea a little further by giving their patients injections of female hormone, with still more beneficial results. They didn't actually cure these far-advanced cases, but they made them a great deal better than they were. Recurrent breast cancer is now widely treated by massive doses of the so-called masculinizing hormones, particularly those of the adrenal gland.

In other types of far-advanced cancer, removing the original growth seems to slow down a great deal the rate of development of the metastatic colonies. Surgeons have seen this demonstrated time and again when they have operated on cancers of the intestine that have spread to the liver. Removing the original growth causes the liver colony to shrink to a marked degree and thus prolongs life.

Yes, cancer can be cured, even in relatively far advanced cases. But it is the early case, the one who comes to treatment while the outlaw cells still remain in the original location, or before the extreme outer barricades of lymph nodes have been breached, that yields the most satisfactory result. And it is to such cases that surgeons are appealing for examination and treatment.

Now let us go back to the cause of cancer, or even before that, to the pre-cause. Changes in the body that may become malignant are called precancerous, and surgeons are trying to teach people to come for examination while the growth is still not malignant or is in the very early stages.

Not that every tumor is cancer, far from it. One class of growth definitely is not malignant, although some of them undoubtedly do turn into cancer later on. These are the benign tumors, localized nests of cells that go on a growing spree of their own at times but are too shy to start invading other cells. Many tumors are of this type. For instance, the lumps that develop in the thyroid gland and appear to cause no trouble are benign tumors of thyroid cells, called adenomas by the surgeon, and goiters by the layman. But these thyroid adenomas aren't as harmless as they seem, for many of them do develop into cancers. Generally speaking, it is better to remove tumors like this before they have a chance to become malignant.

Or consider the lumps of fat that occur here and there from time to time, called lipomas. These are almost always benign tumors; they rarely become cancerous. Benign tumors can cause a lot of trouble, however. Inside the chest, for example, a cyst—which is merely a baglike benign tumor filled with fluid—may start growing and press on vital organs until it interferes with breathing and with the proper functioning of the heart. It doesn't actually invade anything, but it causes trouble by elbowing others out of the way. Surgeons generally advise removal of benign tumors before they actually cause trouble, because of the odd chance that some of them will turn into cancers—as we know some of them do.

Certain other conditions do predispose to cancer. Skin that has been overtreated with radium, X-ray, other types of radiation, or even with ultraviolet and sunlight, tends to develop cancer much more frequently than protected skin. Scars, such as burn scars, are definitely weak spots. Thyroid tumors have already been mentioned. There is always the possibility of a cyst developing a cancer inside itself and rapidly becoming invaded by this unwelcome passenger. Cancer of the liver seems to develop in livers previously damaged by infection, poisoning, or even alcohol.

In short, anything that distorts normal structures may set up in them a liability to cancer. The mere fact of the development of cancer in an organ is *prima facie* evidence that something about the organ wasn't quite normal either in its developing or in its functioning, or that it was damaged in some way.

Even the increased incidence of cancer in old age becomes easily explainable then, for age causes changes from normal in all body cells, changes that apparently predispose to cancer. That is why malignant disease increases so rapidly after fifty, and why the older person has to be at least twice as observant for changes from normal in his own body as the younger individual. In another way, though, age is a beneficial factor, for the older the person, the less severe is liable to be the cancer he may develop, and the more certain the likelihood of a cure.

Heredity in cancer is perhaps the least-understood phase of the whole subject, yet in many ways the most fascinating. Fortunately for man, the mouse has a group of tumors that are easily studied in the laboratory. And, too, the breeding rate is so great that generation after generation can be bred and the heredity factors studied effectively in a short period of time. Several laboratories devoted entirely to cancer research now have mice with unbelievably long family trees, and from them much about cancer has been learned.

It seems perfectly true that cancer, or rather the tendency toward it, can be inherited. Which doesn't mean that because your grandmother had a cancer you are shortly going to die a horrible death. If your grandmother lived to a very ripe old age, there was considerable likelihood that she would develop malignant disease because of age alone. Certain families do show definitely recurring strains of cancer, occurring in the same region in generation after generation. Thus in mice strains can be developed in which the likelihood of cancer approaches 100 per cent.

Some evidence tends to indicate that part of the answer to the cause of cancer may lie in the vast, unexplored field of those ultramicroscopic disease agents that we call viruses, which cause such well-known minor calamities as measles, mumps, and tobacco mosaic disease. In this work, thus far limited to animal experimentation, such a virus has been isolated and found to cause constantly recurring malignant tumors in rabbits and mice. Some day an earnest research scientist is going to stumble on the answer to the cause of cancer, and perhaps on a simple cure for it at the same time. For a long time it looked as if there would never be an answer to the disease poliomyelitis, but the Salk vaccine now promises to control that disease and one day eradicate it completely.

Meanwhile there is no need to throw up our hands in despair because we don't yet know why cancer occurs. Early treatment, adequate treatment, is still good treatment—and it will cure cancer. Let us examine a few of the more common types of malignant growth in order to evaluate the place of surgery in treating this disease.

Cures in cancer are usually stated in terms of five years without evidence of recurrence, ordinarily called "five-year cures." It is not entirely true that a "five-year cure" is a permanent cure, but the statistics vary so little from five to ten years that generally five years can be accepted as meaning the cancer was almost certainly successfully removed in the early stages, before metastasis had occurred.

Cancers of the skin are fairly frequent, particularly with advancing age, and yield perhaps the best results of all cancers to surgery and radiation. Generally speaking, cancers of the skin are either basal-cell cancers, the ulcers that develop on the faces of older people and are called "rodent ulcers" because of their tendency to gnaw gradually at the skin of the nose, face, or eyelids, or the more superficial type called epidermoid, or squamous cell.

Basal-cell cancers are easily killed by X-ray and radium. Since they rarely enter the blood stream by metastasis, they offer the best prognosis; the cure rate averages about 74 per cent with ordinary methods of treatment by radiation or surgical removal. For epidermoid cancers, which tend to spread somewhat faster than the basal-cell type, the cure rate runs from 50 to 60 per cent of all cases. In those treated early, the results are much better.

All cancer results inevitably include people who die of some intercurrent disease but who are usually listed as deaths from cancer. When these are excluded from the final figures, the average survival rate reported by some clinics rises to 85 per cent. Interestingly enough, the normal death rate of all cases in the five-year period in this older age group is about 25 per cent. The obvious corollary is that a person who has a face cancer properly treated has as good a chance of living as he would have anyway, which isn't entirely true but is close enough to let ride.

Cancers of the breast are relatively frequent—for cancers.

Fortunately in no condition has the surgical treatment been so well worked out and so well standardized. Several decades ago famed pioneer surgeon William H. Halstead, of Johns Hopkins, devised the operation that has become standard throughout the world. It consists of removal of the breast and the areas into which breast cancers commonly spread, the muscles beneath the breast, the skin over the tumor, and the lymph vessels and nodes in the breast area. In competent hands, this operation has a mortality rate that is negligible, probably not as high as from appendectomy, and the results are extremely gratifying.

Here again final results depend on early diagnosis, but tumors of the breast are easily examined and can be found before they have advanced very far. There is almost no excuse for an inoperable cancer of the breast. The woman who waits to consult a surgeon about her breast tumor until it is large, ulcerating, with lymph nodes involved, and probably a lump of metastatic cancer in her bones or elsewhere, has committed suicide almost as certainly as if she had blown out her brains with a pistol.

Whether or not to use radiation with surgery in the treatment of breast cancer has been a subject of active, sometimes vehement, discussion in medical societies for years. Gradually now the wheat is being sifted from the chaff and most surgeons have agreed on a policy of treatment. Generally it can be said that neither X-ray nor radium is a substitute for surgery, and the same is true of the isotopes more recently developed as a result of the discoveries in atomic energy. This truth cannot be emphasized too strongly.

In her desire to escape operation, largely due to a misunderstanding of the procedure itself and what is accomplished, the luckless patient may seek radiation before surgery, without consulting a surgeon and, unfortunately, find someone—not a qualified radiologist—who will give it to her with the assurance that a cure will shortly follow. It is true that the growth will shrink, may seem to disappear, but the patient is living in a fool's paradise. Unless the cancer is removed by the surgeon's scalpel it always recurs, usually meaning a hopeless prognosis.

Surgery and radiation do have a place together, a large proportion of cancer surgeons agree, but it is just that—together. Some surgeons prefer radiation before operation, more of them afterward. But the growth *must be removed by an operation*. And most cancer surgeons agree again, the extent of the operation should not be influenced in any way by the fact that the patient either has had radiation or will have it after operation.

And now the results of breast-cancer surgery. If operated on while the outlaw cells are still confined to the breast, five-year survivals have been reported in from 55 to 80 per cent of the cases. Involvement of the neighboring lymph nodes, specifically those of the armpit, lowers the survival rate to a low 45 per cent, an unanswerable argument against waiting to see whether the lump is growing.

Before leaving the breast, a word about breast tumors. It is a safe bet for a woman to consider every breast tumor a reason to consult a competent physician. It is perfectly true that in most lumps in the breast experienced surgeons can determine from the examination alone whether there is a cancer. But these same experienced cancer surgeons rarely call a lump benign in a woman of the cancer age and let it go at that.

A much better principle and one stressed by cancer specialists is that the only certain way to tell a cancer is under the microscope. The general procedure is to remove the lump—local anesthesia or Pentothal make this no more unpleasant than having a tooth fixed—and have it examined microscopically by a competent pathologist. If it is obviously benign, the patient doesn't have to stay in the hospital overnight in most cases. If it is cancer, it has been diagnosed at the earliest possible stage, making a cure extremely probable by immediate removal of the breast.

It is a safe maxim that in the breast, any lump is cancer until the microscope says No.

Perhaps no cancer treatment arouses more misapprehension than that of the digestive tract. Diagnosis of cancer involving the gastrointestinal tract by no means indicates an early demise. The results are in many ways very encouraging, and surgical science is working always to improve the chance of surviving operation—now amazingly good. For example, in some of our leading clinics the operative death rate in resection of the stomach for cancer is now considerably less than five per cent. Until very recently, the mortality rate from appendicitis over the country was no better. Mortality following operation on the rectum, another frequent location for cancer, is little, if any, higher in the better surgical clinics of the country.

Cancer of the stomach is difficult to diagnose. For that reason the number of cases that can be operated on when they present themselves to the surgeon is usually limited, averaging about half of them. The symptoms of stomach cancer are not clear-cut, although a gastric hemorrhage in a person in the cancer age is a demand bid for careful investigation, as is prolonged indigestion, especially with the absence of hydrochloric acid from the gastric analysis of stomach contents.

Of particular interest to the sufferer from stomach ulcer—gastric, not duodenal—is the occurrence of cancer in gastric ulcers. Based on studies at Massachusetts General Hospital, Boston surgeons Arthur W. Allen and Claude E. Welch recommend immediate surgery in gastric ulcers diagnosed in patients over fifty; in ulcers over 2.5 centimeters (roughly an inch) in diameter; if there is no free hydrochloric acid; in ulcers on the greater curvature, the bottom part of the stomach; or in chronic ulcers that do not heal. They conclude that gastric ulcer—again not duodenal, for duodenal ulcer rarely turns to cancer—is basically a surgical lesion and should be removed when there is any question. More and more surgeons are coming to advise resection in gastric ulcers that do not heal after short periods of treatment.

One adjunct to diagnosis has contributed greatly to determining the true nature of stomach conditions. This is the gastroscope. An ingenious combination of a straight metal tube with a flexible rubber section containing many small lenses, the gastroscope can be passed into the stomach with little discomfort and enables the observer to look around a corner, so to speak, and visualize almost the entire stomach cavity. With the gastroscope it is possible to watch the healing of ulcers from week to week, to sight suspicious changes in the edges warning of the development of cancer.

Treatment of stomach cancer is by removing a large portion

of the stomach, sometimes the entire organ, along with the neighboring lymph nodes. The small intestine is then connected to the cut end of the stomach or esophagus. An ingenious double-passage tube enables the surgeon to keep the stomach empty following operation, at the same time putting liquid food into the intestine below the operative area. In cancers that are not too far advanced to permit resection, cures have been obtained in as high as 30 per cent of the cases. If diagnosed early, before the neighboring lymph nodes are involved, the figure ranges from 45 to 60 per cent.

Cancer of the small intestine is rare.

Surgery of the colon advanced tremendously with the discovery of new sulfonamides, such as Sulfasuxadine and sulfaguanidine, whereby it was possible practically to sterilize the normally germ-teeming intestinal contents. With the antibiotic drugs, coupled with the new knowledge of shock and prevention of postoperative complications by means of the Miller-Abbott tube and plasma injections and transfusions, operative mortality from colon surgery has gone down rapidly. In many clinics it is lower than the mortality over the country from appendicitis.

Colon tumors are usually bleeding tumors and call attention to their presence by the appearance of blood in the stools. In the first part of the colon, located on the right side, the bleeding may not be immediately apparent and the patient often becomes markedly anemic, a symptom that automatically makes a cancer surgeon suspect cancer in an older person. On the left side, the bleeding is brighter in color, therefore more noticeable. Diagnosis is not difficult with X-ray by means of injection of barium into the colon.

Resection of the colon is normally performed in two ways. First is by removal of the tumor and a direct rejoining of the intestine by sutures, called anastomosis. The other method, equally successful, is called the Mickulicz operation and consists essentially of pulling the bowel containing the tumor out through the incision and cutting off and removing the tumor. The bowel is then allowed to drain through the wound for a short time, after which the connection is re-established and the wound is closed. Results with the two operations seem equally good, but the primary anastomosis is becoming the operation of choice because of the protection against infection provided by the newer drug discoveries.

Five-year survival rates after removal of the right colon range from 50 to 70 per cent, on the left side about 40 per cent, the difference being in the type of tumor that develops. On the right side, cancers tend to protrude into the bowel itself, invading the wall late in their course. Tumors on the left side obstruct early and spread more directly.

Cancer of the rectum, a rather frequent type, is probably responsible for much of the pessimism with which bowel cancers are generally regarded. This arises because the operative removal often results in a colostomy. Results of operation generally give about 45 per cent cures. Many surgeons are now beginning to believe that in many rectal cases it is not necessary to end up with a colostomy, and possibly the wider adoption of this viewpoint may remove much of the patient's horror of the procedure. Fortunately, cancer of the rectum can be diagnosed early because the symptom of hemorrhage calls attention to its presence and visualization is simple by examination and with the proctoscope.

In the female reproductive tract, a fairly common type of cancer occurs, that of the uterus. Two types of growth occur here, one in the fundus on the top of the uterus, the other in the cervix. Fundus cancer is generally treated by surgery with or without radiation. In early cases, cures may run as high as 70 per cent or more.

Cancer of the cervix, the most frequent form in the female generative tract, is commonly treated by radium, although many surgeons believe that in early cases operative removal of the entire uterus yields best results. Cures here run as high as 63 per cent, averaging 40 per cent or more.

Within the past decade a new field of cancer has been attacked surgically, cancer of the lung. Long regarded as a hopeless area for malignant disease, the lung, thanks to modern operative technique, can now be removed safely. Thousands of cases have demonstrated that curability rates here average close to 50 per cent. The operative mortality, once almost forbiddingly high, is small now in skilled hands.

At present, a considerable controversy is raging over the question of whether smoking leads to lung cancer. Cancer specialists of considerable experience and authority maintain that it does, while others of equal accomplishment stoutly disagree. Undoubtedly the truth will come out in a few years, and it may very well be that something used in preparing tobacco for cigarette smoking will ultimately turn out to be the causative agent in the undeniably marked increase of lung cancer over the past several decades.

Another new field of cancer surgery, too, is the pancreas, which is now being attacked successfully all over the world.

A new surgical specialty has sprung up, cancer surgery. The surgeons are trained in the techniques of removal of all types of malignant disease. Because of their specialization, their results will steadily improve, in lives saved, both at operation and after operation.

There is little need for pessimism in cancer, but there is a real need for a new consciousness on the part of those approaching the cancer age, a consciousness that only if they present themselves early and regularly for examination and treatment can the fight against cancer be carried out.

Surgery cures cancer—the figures prove it.

23.

WHY SURGERY IS EXPENSIVE

---

*Good surgery quite costly or entirely free—
Finances of hospitals—Charity work by surgeons
—The cost of making a surgeon—Surgeons' in-
comes—How to locate a good surgeon—Clinics—
Hospitals*

Good surgery is either quite costly or entirely free. Even
more paradoxical, whether paid for or free, surgical care is
frequently given by the same surgeon, though working under
vastly different circumstances.

As an example, a tailor from the slums goes to a famous
hospital and medical school, entering by the clinic door.
When it is determined that he is not financially able to pay
for service, he is admitted to the outpatient department,
where his case is worked up by a medical student or intern
and presented to the professor of surgery. Examination shows
that the sick man has a tumor of the lung which should be
removed. He is admitted to the hospital and the operation
performed by the most expert surgeon at the institution. The
patient receives all necessary blood transfusions and special
treatments as a matter of course.

The same afternoon, the same professor of surgery may
operate for exactly the same condition on the president of
a railroad. His fee may very well be $5,000, and several
thousand more may go for hospital charges. Both patients get
equal treatment; both get the same result.

Admittedly this is an extreme case, but the same principles
hold true in the economic applications of medical care everywhere. Good lifesaving surgery, with all the adjuncts that

modern science has given to this business of saving lives, usually costs more than the average man can afford to pay— if he pays for it himself. Is this because the doctors and hospitals are getting rich? A glance at the record settles that question.

Very few hospitals in this country pay their own way from bills paid by patients, although the financial condition of hospitals in general has been tremendously improved by the widespread adoption of various forms of hospital insurance by large sections of the population. Many large medical centers, particularly those connected with medical schools, are supported entirely by charity. Others, small private institutions, often run by doctor groups, have a deficit that these doctors are willing to cover because of the advantage of having their patients in the same building as their offices, with adequate facilities to practice medicine and surgery the way they want to practice it. In between lies a great group of hospitals whose losses are financed by churches, cities, philanthropic groups, and numberless other methods.

Costs of hospital care, too, are increasing as science puts ever newer weapons into the hands of the doctors who are fighting death and who demand that these adjuncts be made available to their patients. Special instruments and apparatus must be present in a well-run hospital; to name but a few, fluoroscopes, X-rays, electrocardiographs, metabolism machines, allergy-testing materials, oscillometers for testing blood-vessel pulsations, thermocouples for measuring changes in skin temperature, a freezing microtome to cut instantly sections of a tissue removed in the operating room and return a diagnosis of cancer or benign tumor while the anesthetist keeps the patient asleep, special anesthetic aids such as cyclopropane, oxygen, and oxygen tents—and a thousand other items, all costing a great deal of money.

Insurance companies know that it takes about the same administrative cost to pay a small claim as a large one. In the same way it takes about as many bookkeepers, business managers, and secretaries to collect small hospital bills as large ones. Nursing staffs must be kept complete. Ambulances, if operated by the hospital, have running expenses and depreciation. Laundry becomes a formidable item when bed linen is changed every day, oftener when patients are very ill. A staff of interns and residents must be kept, housed, fed, clothed, and sometimes paid. The hospital goes on eating up resources whether half full or empty. A national magazine reported the operating expenses of one of the largest medical centers at more than five million dollars a year. Only 68 per cent of its income came from patients' fees; the rest was derived from donations or from investments.

The 1942 average daily operating cost for general hospitals in New York City was reported by *Medical Economics* as $7.21 per patient. Daily costs of smaller hospitals averaging several hundred beds were close to $6 per patient. Columbia-Presbyterian Medical Center was reported as having an average daily cost of $10.28 per patient, with a daily income from patients averaging $6.75 per patient. Detailed present day figures are not available but price rises have roughly doubled those quoted and sometimes made them even larger.

Hundreds of similar examples could be given to show that hospitals in general make no profit and usually operate at a loss. Medical care is expensive, then, but not because hospitals are making large profits.

What of the surgeons' fees?

If surgical care is costly, is it because surgeons charge exorbitant fees and profiteer at the expense of patients who are able to pay?

Most surgeons would admit that if they were paid proportionately for all their operations, the individual cost could be lowered a great deal. In every large city will be found many surgeons who devote from a third to half their time to working in charity hospitals from which they receive nothing. In most cases this is a labor of love, the medical man's traditional privilege of serving humanity by giving his services to those who cannot pay. Undeniably there are certain advantages to the surgeon also.

The prestige of position on the charity-hospital staff is worth a great deal, since these positions are rarely handed out to any but those of excellent professional qualifications. Add to this the facilities for research, available otherwise to only a small number of relatively poorly paid full-time teachers in medical schools, and the advantage of being able to polish operative technique by performing many operations of the same type. There can be no question that his charity work benefits a surgeon in many ways, but it does not help pay his office expenses.

The cost of surgical training and experience must always be counted into any evaluation of the surgeon's right to charge relatively high fees. The average man finishing college has completed his education and is ready to make a living. The would-be surgeon is merely at the beginning. Facing him first are four years of medical school. Tuition at these schools now averages $1,000 or more a year. Add to this living expenses and the cost for a year of medical education usually runs a minimum of $2,000 and is more generally $2,500 or more. So strenuous, too, is the medical course that rarely is any medical student able to engage in a profitable part-time activity.

At the end of his medical course, the doctor has a cost above college expenses of at least eight to ten thousand dollars. Had he been working at any other occupation, even the relatively low-paid profession of teaching school, he would have made at least that much more, putting his total loss for the four years at a minimum of eighteen to twenty thousand dollars, without any advantages of seniority.

Were the surgeon then ready to practice his profession, the outlay would not be disproportionate to his final expected income, but actually he is not a surgeon at all when he finishes medical school. As presently organized, surgical training actually begins only after graduation from medical school and continues for a minimum of five years, if he is to be certified as a specialist by the American Board of Surgery, the certification board for the field of general surgery, or one of the other specialty boards. Nowhere more than in surgery is the aphorism more true that a craftsman must first serve as an apprentice, and as an apprentice he receives no pay. If a doctor intends to perfect himself in the field of surgery, he must then plan on allocating at least five years to developing skill and ability in his chosen field, after graduating from medical school.

Five years means a loss from probable income, even again as a teacher, of from $15,000 to $20,000. Rarely is the surgeon in training able to afford anything more expensive than term insurance during these years when he serves successively as a hospital intern, assistant resident, and finally resident surgeon. All of which means that at the point when he finishes the five years' surgical training, nine years after graduation from college, and is ready to begin earning, he is nine years older from an insurance standpoint than the college graduate, with the consequent increase in rates.

In those five years' training, the embryo surgeon does have some income. Usually the first year he gets nothing but food, clothing, and room, and furnishes his spending money himself. By the fourth year he may work up to a salary of $100 per month, rarely more, often less. If he plans to become a full-time teacher of surgery in a medical school, several more years of low-paid training are required before he realizes that ambition, and he never really makes any large annual income.

When the surgeon finally steps out of the hospital, ready to practice his specialty, he is roughly twenty to thirty thousand dollars or more in the red over what he would have been had he started teaching or some similar occupation at the end of college.

Suppose, for example, he had studied engineering instead of medicine. Graduating with a Ph. D. in engineering three years after finishing college, he can almost pick his job at a starting salary of from $750 to $900 per month. The surgeon going into practice, on the other hand, must equip an office, probably costing a minimum of $2,000, usually three to five thousand. And in the first year, if he is lucky, he loses no more than $2,000. In the second year he begins to break even.

Now that he is financially on his own feet with his own office, how can a patient go about finding this qualified surgeon in any town or city? The best answer lies, of course, in letting the family doctor pick out the surgeon best qualified to handle the particular problem. Unfortunately, the family doctor is fading rather rapidly out of the picture, too.

With a shifting population, modern methods of transportation, and the tendency of people to crowd together in cities, medicine is being practiced more and more by clinics. Or people go directly to the specialist who treats whatever it is they think is wrong with them. Doctors agree that this is the poorest way of all to choose a doctor, but the American way is to shoot for the top at the beginning and hope for the best.

Coming into a strange city, probably the poorest way to choose a doctor is on the advice of the neighbors around you, the drugstore man at the corner, or across the grocer's counter. One simple way is to pick up the phone and call the nearest doctor's office. Ask his secretary for the name of the president or secretary of the local medical society.

Practically every county in the country has such a society. Ask the county-society official for the names of a number of doctors who treat your particular condition. Unless you are absolutely certain of your diagnosis, from previous experience, ask for internists, specialists in internal medicine, or competent general practitioners. The officer will in almost every case give you the names of several men, and you can feel confident that any of them will be able to take care of you.

Another method is to consult the largest hospital in the city and ask the name of the chief of whatever department in which you think your complaint lies. If there is a large charity hospital in the city, especially a county or city hospital, ask for the name of the chief of service in the specialty you are interested in. As far as surgery is concerned, he is almost certain to be one of the top specialists in that field. If unable to take care of you himself, he can refer you to a capable specialist, usually one of the younger men.

Still another method is to consult the city library in your locality. Ask to see the Directory of Medical Specialties. If the library does not have it, the local hospital usually does. Listed here are all the certified specialists in the country. A certified specialist has appeared before a national board of experts, who have decided that he is fully qualified to practice his specialty. You cannot possibly go wrong in choosing him.

If the specialist directory is not available, most libraries and practically all hospitals have a copy of the American Medical Directory. Published by the American Medical Association, this large volume lists up-to-date information on every doctor practicing in the United States and some neighboring countries. Look first for the state and then city or county you are in, then move down the list of names.

Names listed in heavy type are Fellows of the American Medical Association, the first step in choosing recognized by physicians.

If you are searching only for surgeons, seek next for the letter S after a doctor's name. That means he's primarily a surgeon; if the S is followed by a star, that means he limits his practice to surgery. A small set of numbers after his name will tell you from what medical school he graduated and when, by referring to a key to the abbreviation spaced at frequent intervals in the directory before the listings for each state. To find a certified specialist, follow the list of S-marked names down until the key *A.B. 12* appears. This means that the surgeon has been certified by the American Board of Surgery, the highest qualifying board in the country in general surgery. Other numbers following the abbreviations *A.B.* designate the certification in other specialties.

Only the larger cities will have surgeons certified by the American Board of Surgery, since only a few thousand surgeons have been thus certified. For this reason, another method of picking out a capable surgeon in a strange city is needed. Locating again the name of a doctor after whose name the letter S appears, you will see just after the S, an *A* followed by several numbers in small type. *A28* means that this surgeon is a Fellow of the American College of Surgeons and therefore recognized as a capable surgeon by the officers of that great organization. Again you can safely stop and call one of the surgeons designated by this number.

If no Fellow of the American College of Surgeons appears in the city, take the doctors who list S and a star, or S after their names. These men are surgeons, recognized as such in their community.

In locating physicians with other specialties refer to the "Key to Specialties" listed before each state in the directory. They include all the medical specialties and give you at a glance the qualifications of each doctor so listed.

In most cases, unless a specialist is needed, a doctor from the directory can be called. Do not be misled by the term doctor. Not all so-called "doctors" are M.D.'s, but all M.D.'s are doctors. In a strange city you can't afford to pick anything but the best.

The American Medical Directory not only lists doctors, it lists hospitals. When in doubt about the hospital to go to, look at the listing of hospitals in front of each state. These are recognized hospitals. If marked with a star they have been approved for internship by the Council on Medical Education and Hospitals of the A.M.A. A small black cross means approval for residencies in specialties. Both designations are complete assurance that it is a well-run and competent hospital, to which you can safely entrust yourself. If not designated by these symbols, the hospital is still likely to be satisfactory, so long as it is listed in the directory.

24.

MEDICINE IN THE ATOMIC AGE

Almost complete control of medical diseases—Increase in degenerative diseases—A population of older people—New medical specialty, geriatrics—New discoveries to be expected—Increasing importance of endocrine glands, hormones—The question of socialized medicine—Hospital insurance—Group clinics

The first few years following the end of World War II saw many doctors formerly in uniform returning to civil life. This change meant considerable hardship to many of them. New adjustments had to be made, new equipment bought, for already many instruments and apparatus in use before the war were obsolete. New contacts with the public had to take place. In general, the doctor returning from the armed forces was in almost the same position that he had been when he had started practice.

Many doctors were in military positions calling for little professional work. In no walk of life is it so true as in medicine that a few months away from his tools dulls the skill of the workman. These doctors needed refresher courses in medicine and surgery; many whose training had been interrupted wished to go on through additional training, and others who had not yet prepared themselves for specialties wished to do so. Hardships, financial and otherwise, were inevitable in spite of the prosperity that followed World War II.

With new antibiotic drugs being discovered practically every day, infectious diseases caused by microbes and viruses have sharply declined in the past decade. Death rates in recent years have shown a sharp drop; there has been, in fact, an almost unbelievable decline in deaths from infectious diseases. It is not at all improbable that the next decade will see a continuation of this trend. Widespread prophylaxis by antibiotic and other drugs against meningitis, sore throat, rheumatic fever, scarlet fever, and the rest of the great group of diseases caused by the ubiquitous streptococcus blazed a trail for more complete control of these infections in the future. The Army's experience with meningitis is a striking example of what can be done to curb scourges like this.

Meningitis, doctors have long known, can be divided into two stages, the early period of blood-stream infection with the meningococcus, called meningococcemia, and the late stage of true invasion of the tissues around the brain and spinal cord by the deadly microbes. Rarely in civil life is the disease diagnosed in the early stages when it is most susceptible to attack by drug treatment.

In the armed forces, with troops under close medical observation at all times to prevent epidemics, many cases of meningococcic infection were diagnosed and treated before actual meningitis ever developed. An excellent example of this occurred in a series reported from a Southern camp. At this post there were more than a hundred cases under treatment for meningococcal infection, with a mortality rate of less than three per cent.

In the same county there were eight civilian cases of meningitis, four of whom died—a mortality rate of 50 per cent.

Meningitis, once diagnosed properly, yields rapidly to treatment with sulfadiazine and other drugs. At the time of this outbreak, sulfadiazine was freely used but penicillin was only beginning to be used and was not available for treatment of anything except special diseases. Before the tale of chemotherapy is finally told, particularly with so many new drugs of the antibiotic group being discovered, many other diseases will be found to yield as rapidly as does this once dreadful infection of meningitis. But it is still better to prevent the disease wherever possible than to wait until it develops before treating it.

The way to that end, with meningitis—and pointing out a new trail for other diseases, too—was shown in the spring of

1943 and reported in the *Military Surgeon* by Lieutenant Colonel Joseph F. Painton, of the Army Medical Corps.

From April 27, 1943, until May 21 at a large Army Air Force training center, cases of meningococcemia were admitted at the rate of one a day. This is a frequent occurrence when great numbers of raw troops are brought together for the first time, with many disease carriers thus placed in contact with the whole group. It was decided in this camp that a meningitis epidemic of a dangerous nature was on the point of developing and that drastic prophylaxis was indicated.

On that date the entire enlisted personnel of this large training center, about 18,000 persons, were started on sulfadiazine prophylaxis. Each person received about five grams of the drug in eighteen hours, considerably less than the amount ordinarily given in twenty-four hours of treatment with sulfadiazine and later shown to be a much larger dose than necessary for satisfactory prophylaxis against meningitis.

The results of this experiment in preventing disease settled for all time the question of the value of drug prophylaxis and pointed the way to a possible complete eradication of the disease as a major cause of death in epidemic form. In the eight weeks following the administration of the one-day sulfadiazine protection:

No case of meningitis or meningococcemia developed among any of the personnel who had been "diazined."

Other side effects of this experiment were equally startling. No case of scarlet fever developed in the eight-week period, and the incidence of respiratory infections was cut in half over the ensuing nine days. Similar experiments at large Naval bases had shown that the rate of respiratory infections, septic sore throats, and similar illnesses could be materially reduced by relatively small doses of sulfadiazine.

But if a near miracle has been accomplished in lowering mortality rates from infectious diseases, no such happy prospect has appeared in regard to the so-called degenerative diseases, those that occur with age. Actuarial figures show that the United States, more than any other nation, is rapidly becoming a land of older people. The reason for this is quickly obvious. Lower the incidence of infectious diseases and the fall in death rates from this source naturally increases the life span of the population. Figures show a steady increase in life expectancy over many years, but along with this has gone a sharp rise in the degenerative diseases.

This doesn't mean that cancer, diabetes, and heart trouble, to name the three greatest degenerative diseases, are on an actual percentage increase, although there is considerable evidence that heart afflictions, particularly coronary heart disease, do seem to be increasing with the tensions of modern civilized living. What it does mean is that the population is gradually encompassing a greater and greater percentage of people in the age group in which these diseases occur. Thus it is inevitable that death rates will rise from these causes and will keep on rising unless some great catastrophe should decimate the older sections of the population.

The great problem of the medical profession is to find ways to combat these degenerative diseases and to reverse the trend. Already much has been done to control diabetes and heart trouble, to prolong the lives of those who suffer from them, and in the case of cancer, to effect a complete cure.

Age is being attacked by an entirely new medical specialty called geriatrics. Interestingly enough, much has been done to combat the effects of old age. Obviously a person's numerical age cannot be influenced, but his functional age can, considered in terms of body and mental activity.

Science stands on the threshold of a vast field of unexplored material about the endocrine glands, those powerful little factories producing the hormones that largely control body function. The startling accomplishments of ACTH and cortisone are evidence of what has been and still is to be accomplished in this field. The Sunday-supplement picture of a man kept always youthful by a daily tablet from the medicine cabinet may eventually be closer to the truth than any of us believes.

The harnessing of atomic power in the great laboratories of the Atomic Energy Commission has seen a new branch of medicine come into being, that having to do with radioactive substances, notably the elements called isotopes. And here the promise of the future seems great.

Radium has for many years been an important weapon in the fight against cancer, yet radium is extremely expensive.

Cobalt, made radioactive in the atomic furnace, can now be produced at a cost of roughly one-thousandth that of radium. In addition, its effects can be far more effectively concentrated than radium. Eventually, it seems, cobalt may well supplant natural radium for this purpose.

Internally, several of the radioactive isotopes seem to hold considerable promise in medical and surgical treatment. One, at least, in indicated cases, is an effective substitute for surgery, namely the radioactive isotope of iodine, I^{131}, in hyperthyroidism.

Prior to World War II, the most effective treatment of hyperthyroidism—a strange and little-understood condition in which the thyroid gland begins to overact and upsets the metabolism of the entire body—was surgery. But results were often erratic, and operation dangerous. Drugs of the thiouracil type helped control hyperthyroidism, particularly as a prelude to operation, as did X-ray therapy. Iodine, in the body, is concentrated in the thyroid gland and has long been used in treating this condition, again particularly as a prelude to surgery. Radioactive iodine, however, seemed to offer three distinct advantages: it could be taken internally, it was concentrated in the gland, and it would have the same effect on it as X-rays.

I^{131}, the radioactive isotope of iodine, has proved remarkably effective in treating simple hyperthyroidism, where there are no nodules to add the risk of later cancer formation. One dose, taken simply by mouth, effects a cure in a large proportion of cases of simple hyperthyroidism, a much easier and more effective treatment than surgery ever was.

In thyroid cancer, radioactive iodine helps control distant metastases, by concentrating radiation into inaccessible parts of the body, where the malignant tissue has spread. I^{131} has also proved valuable in thyroid diagnosis, where determinations of the percentage of the radioactive iodine concentrated in the thyroid gland seems to give an even better indication of thyroid function than determination of basal metabolism, the time-honored test.

Radioactive phosphorus, P^{32}, has proved to be of tremendous value in treating a rather obscure medical condition, polycythemia vera, and in some forms of the blood cancer called leukemia.

Radioactive gold, Au^{198}, is of great value when injected into the chest cavity of advanced cancer cases in which fluid formation causes great discomfort. When methods of placing radioactive gold directly into other tumors are worked out, its value may be considerably broadened.

No doubt other radioactive materials will find expanded uses in medicine, but they seem unlikely to replace surgery in indicated conditions, although as adjuncts in cancer surgery they will no doubt find wider and wider application.

In another field, a striking discovery of recent years, the beneficial effect of the pituitary and adrenal-cortex hormones, ACTH and cortisone, also is helpful as an adjunct to surgical treatment. Notably is this true in deep shock, such as has been described in connection with severe burns, in which the beneficial effect of these "wonder hormones" may be lifesaving. In addition, their use to supplement antibiotics in fighting infection will undoubtedly be as important in surgery as it has already become in strictly medical practice.

Enabling people to live longer and thus increasing the number of older people in the population carries with it a definite liability on the economic side. The inevitable trend is toward a society in which more and more people depend on others for their sustenance. It is perfectly true that new methods of manufacture, the possible release of hitherto undreamed of sources of energy from atomic disruption, and the many other discoveries that resulted from the tremendous speeding up of research during wartime will make working hours shorter and incomes higher. It is also true that advances in medical science will keep a greater number of people at work at any given time. Balanced against this is the necessity to give the aging population food and clothing and more medical care.

How will this increased need be satisfied? How will its economics be arranged? Where does the answer to the cost of medical care lie?

Some would find it in socialized medicine under various names. In England it is called National Health Insurance, in the United States Compulsory Health Insurance. While England has succumbed to the lure of something for nothing, Americans are traditionally reluctant to hand over any more of their freedom to the government and have resisted the various bills introduced into nearly every Congress to bring about government medical care. Meanwhile, Americans have been doing something about this problem themselves, by the traditional method of working together against a common threat.

The period following the end of World War II has seen a tremendous advance in various forms of voluntary health insurance, notably the one sponsored by the doctors themselves, Blue Cross and Blue Shield. Private insurance companies have also widely popular plans. Under the various voluntary plans, hospital costs and a portion at least of medical and surgical costs can be covered by insurance, at a cost the average worker is quite able to pay. It does not seem at all fantastic to assume that the day is not far off when everyone, not compelled by financial lack to accept care by municipal, county, state, or national government agencies, can protect himself by insurance from medical costs.

Admittedly, a medical disaster such as a long and serious illness or a costly operation could bankrupt even the moderately affluent. Fortunately, even that unlikely eventuality can be avoided through a new plan of what might be called Medical Disaster Insurance. Under it, the first $500 of medical costs, covering hospital, surgeon, special treatments, etc., are paid by the insured out of his regular hospital insurance. Of all costs beyond $500, in one plan that is an example of all, 75 per cent is paid by the company up to $7,500 for each person insured. Thus, for a reasonable premium, a family can be protected against the sometimes disastrous costs of a severe illness.

Meanwhile, more and more doctors are coming to believe that a streamlining is vitally necessary for the present methods of bringing medical knowledge and skill to those who are sick, if we are to be saved from a revolution that may destroy much of the advance made in medical care, should any sort of an economic backset occur. Experiments in various forms of socialism are always much more frequent in times of economic depression, and often changes are made in established procedure that are difficult to alter once the economy has re-adjusted itself, in spite of obvious defects.

The ideal method of streamlining medical care seems to lie in what doctors call a group clinic. What is this concept and what does it mean?

Group clinics are not new. There has been a steadily rising incidence of group formations among doctors from year to year. In spite of this, there were for many years objections among the rank and file of medical men to the idea that doctors could work in groups as effectively as they could as individuals. But the growth of medical science over the years has made such a trend inevitable.

Just as schools have progressed from the frontier concept of a one-room schoolhouse, taught by one teacher who was a jack-of-all-trades, to the great consolidated schools of today in which each teacher is a specialist, so specialization in medicine has become an accepted fact. So vast is the scope of medical knowledge now that no single man can encompass it entirely. Doctors, if they are to bring their patients the highest in medical knowledge and skill, have had to limit their practice to acquire the knowledge available in one field.

When doctors began to specialize, it became inevitable that they would tend to gravitate toward groups where the sum of medical knowledge could be made available to the sick person with a minimum of delay and duplication of effort. Realizing this, a few far-sighted physicians began to form specialist groups many years ago. The growth of such organizations as the Mayo Clinic, the Lahey Clinic, and the many university teaching centers scattered about the country indubitably shows the wisdom and very necessity of this concept.

Nor does grouping specialists mean only a concentration of medical knowledge. It is a far more economical way of working as far as the patient is concerned. A patient going from one doctor to another must inevitably pay for duplication of laboratory work, examinations, X-rays, and all the many adjuncts that modern medicine must have to work effectively. Concentrated in one place, these adjuncts are more effectively used, at considerably less expense to the patient.

Those who do not like group clinics object that the examination and treatment of the patient becomes an assembly-line process, but patients who have been treated in group clinics rarely make such objections. The obvious answer is that the production miracle created by World War II could never have been accomplished without just such methods. It may be equally true that the great increase in medical care necessitated by an aging population, which is also an economic liability, may well demand just such a method.

Usually a group clinic consists of several older men depending on its size and age, and younger doctors in various stages of training and responsibility. Generally, all are specialists. Together they give a thorough coverage of the main fields of medicine.

Financial arrangements differ with groups. Most such organizations, however, find it advantageous to divorce themselves from finances as far as possible. These are handled by a business organization, which charges the patient in proportion to what treatment is necessary and what he can pay. The doctors are thus able to plan the examinations indicated by diagnosis and treatment without considering the expense. Thus the patient automatically gets a complete job, whether he is eventually a profit or loss to the group. Obviously only a certain number of patients can be handled at a loss, unless the clinic is protected by some sort of endowment. Many clinics are thus protected.

The remuneration of the doctors is usually set by mutual consent of the members of the group, with profit shared among them. Rarely is a group successful in which a doctor is remunerated according to the number of patients he treats. The element of financial competition inside the group almost always creates discord. Professional competition is encouraged and stimulates advance in the younger doctor's ability, for only by training younger men can a clinic hope to survive.

But getting back to the patient, what are the benefits to him in group treatment?

A sick person entering an established group clinic does not usually go to any one physician in that group, although he may do so if he wishes. Generally the patient knows that the specialist who knows most about his condition will handle his case eventually. The reason that this supervision is possible is also the greatest advantage of the group.

With the results of many examinations before him, with consultations from other specialists in the group when needed, the most experienced specialist in the field in which the trouble lies can quickly arrive at a diagnosis and indicate the treatment. This treatment will be given either by himself or by someone qualified to give it under his direction. In that way the knowledge and skill accumulated by the specialist over many years can be quickly made available to large numbers of patients, a far larger group than would be possible if he were working alone, personally attending to all the many details of diagnosis and treatment. This economy of effort with the maximum of medical care is undoubtedly the greatest advantage of groups to the patient. Inevitably the patient receives more medical care and better medical care at a lower per-unit cost.

It may be argued that the eventual total cost of group care is greater than individual care because, while the unit cost per examination is lower, more examinations are carried out. This is often perfectly true, but there are definite advantages to this. Routine examinations of the blood, urine, chest X-rays, electrocardiograms, and other commonly performed tests in the group clinics often show up a condition that was not suspected. Treatment can be begun at once, often adding years to the patient's life. Such benefits cannot be measured in dollars and cents.

The main question before the people today seems not to be, Is group medicine better than care by the individual doctor? Actually there seems little doubt about that. Rather it is, Is not group medicine, with some form of prepayment insurance, better than government-furnished medicine from tax funds, with the inevitable waste inherent in such a bureaucracy as would be built up with this system?

As early as 1940, the author proposed in his first novel, *That None Should Die,* a plan of medical care that combined group practice with controlled health insurance. It is reprinted, with slight amendments to cover changing money values, in the following chapter.

25.

A PLAN FOR MEDICAL CARE

Group medicine, with some form of prepayment insurance

In this plan doctors may organize themselves in group clinics according to the population, with the number of the men on the staff, each a competent diagnostician or specialist in some field, depending on the size of the clinic that is justified by the population in that particular area. The American Medical Association will set up minimum standards for the clinics and they must conform to these standards or their franchise will be taken away and given to another more satisfactory organization.

The clinics will take care of all patients in their area who come to them, but patients will not be required to attend any particular clinic, with the exception of the low-income group to be mentioned later. This group, having their medical expenses paid by the state and city governments, with national aid if necessary, must attend the clinic in their locality.

The national and state health departments will continue to function much as now for the prevention of disease, but all treatment must be referred to the clinics. Care of the tuberculous and mentally ill will be handled as at present by the local state and city governments, except that special clinics may be organized similar to private psychiatric clinics today.

The internists in each clinic will be family doctors to their patients in the sense that they will make outside calls wher-

*Reprinted from *That None Should Die* by Frank G. Slaughter, by permission of Doubleday and Company, Inc.

ever necessary, the work usually being delegated to younger men. Ambulance service will be furnished by the clinics, or by private agencies, and all patients sick enough to need close observation will immediately be transferred to the clinic hospital. In sparsely populated areas one or more dressing stations or dispensaries will be maintained at various places by the clinic in that locality, so that the services of a physician will at all times be available to those who need it.

In organizing the clinics, the government will make long-term loans for buying necessary buildings and equipment. These loans will not be grants and must be paid back gradually at a set rate. In some areas it may be necessary to have some direct government subsidy largely because of the sparsity of population. The giving of this subsidy does not carry with it the right of the government to interfere in any way. The state and national medical associations will govern the operation of the clinics entirely.

Payment for medical services as supplied by the clinics will be taken care of as follows:

1. The population of the country will be divided into three income groups:

(a) Low-Income Group—Income less than $2,000 per year for the head of a family or $1,000 per year for a single person. Medical care for this group will be taken care of by the local and state governments by paying the clinics at average cost rates for each patient treated. Patients will be treated in outpatient departments or in the hospitals on the wards. Operations, etc., will be usually done by the house staff under supervision of the specialist of the clinic. All necessary medical care will be given just as if the patient were in higher-income groups. This will entail little more expenditure of tax money, if any, since most of these people are already being cared for by charity hospitals in their areas.

(b) Medium-Income Group—Income from $2,000 to $6,000 per year for heads of families and $1,000 to $3,000 for single persons. Eligible for a system of health insurance collected from their incomes at rates ranging from $5 to $10 for families and $3 per month for a single person.

The insurance fund will be collected and turned over to an insurance commission for each state, consisting of one physician from the state medical association, a member of the United States Public Health Service, and one representative elected by the people. The government has nothing to say about the expenditure of this money. The medical association will work out a system of charges for hospitalization and treatment agreeable to all member clinics. A patient is at liberty to present himself at any clinic in his state and receive necessary treatment of any kind without further charge. The clinics will be reimbursed for this service from the state insurance fund. Persons who do not pay their insurance will not be eligible for treatment under this group.

It is quite possible that for this group some sort of an arrangement with such an existing organization as Blue Cross and Blue Shield could be worked out obviating the duplication of collecting organizations that would otherwise be necessary.

(c) High-Income Group—Income above $3,000 for single and $6,000 for heads of families. These patients must furnish their own medical care as they do now. They will receive whatever accommodations or treatment they wish to pay for at the clinics. They may choose their own clinic and the quality of their accommodations, that is, private room or semi-private. Wards are reserved for low-income group. The patient may arrange insurance himself and then pay the clinic, or an arrangement for the furnishing of medical service similar to that now in use by the Blue Cross and Blue Shield type of insurance organization could be used. In any case the clinic shall have a lien on the insurance paid until any charges assessed against members of this group by the clinics are paid.

Patients in the low-income group are required to attend the clinic in their district at certain specified times, except in case of emergency. Patients in the medium-income group may attend any clinic in their state or, by special arrangement, in another state. Patients in the high-income group may go where they please, since they pay their own way.

2. The clinics will supply medical care for industrial compensation cases when injured at the rates set up by the insurance for the medium-income group. Wherever accident insurance is involved, payment will be made to the clinics taking care of the patients in the usual way.

INDEX

INDEX

Abdominal operations, appendicitis, 58; peritonitis, 58

Abdominal wounds, 65-67; dangers, 65; intestinal feeding, 67

Acacia, use in shock, 14

Acrylic dental splint, 208, 212, 215

ACTH, 5, 9, 200, 207, 252, 254

Addison's Disease, 9

Adrenal cortex, use in shock, 14

Adrenalin, 9, 221

Adrenals, 9, 221

Albumen, control of head pressure, 18

Allen, Arthur W., 237

Aluminum, in skull injuries, 190

Amino acids, 71

Ampulla of Vater, 86

Anastomosis, 88, 117, 238

Anesthesia, ACE, 22; alcohol, 20; atrophine, 27; avertin, 24; barbiturics, 23, 24; caudal injections, 28; in childbirth, 21; chloroform, 20-21, 22; curare, 29; cyclopropane, 23; di-vinyl, 23; ether, 22; ethylene, 23; by injection, 24, 25; morphine, 24, 27; nitrous oxide, 22; novocain, 29; opium, 20; paraldehyde, 24; pentobarbital, 25; Pentothal Sodium, 25, 26, 27; pheno-barbital, 25; positive pressure, 103; refrigeration, 127-130; spinal, 28; thiopentobarbital, 25; tribromoethanol, 24; trimethaphan camphorsulfonate, 29

Aneurysm, formation of, 121-122; operation, 122

Anoxemia, see Oxygen, lack

Antibiotics, 32-43; Aureomycin, 42; chloromycetin, 42; penicillin, 33-43; sulfanilamide, 36, 37; sulfapyridine, 38; sulfathiazole, 39; sulfadiazine, 39; streptomycin, 42; Terramycin, 42

Appendicitis, 58, 59, 68; operations, 59; ice packs, 128

Aristotle, 21

Arteriosclerosis, with refrigeration anesthesia, 128; gangrenous, 131

Arteriovenous aneurysm, 122-126

Arteriovenous fistula, 117, 123

Ashcroft, Major P. B., 168

Au^{198}, 254

Aureomycin, 42

Baer, William S., 44

Balke, Clarence W., 191

Banting, Sir Frederick, 84

Barbiturics, as anesthesia, 23, 24

Beck, Claude, 3, 113-114

Bile, formation of, 72, 74, 75; use of, 70

Blair, Vilray P., 210

Blalock, Alfred, 110, 111, 198

Blood, banks, 66, 206; clotting, 74, 102; substitutes, 19; transfusions, 14-15

Blood clotting, prevention of, citrate solution, 4; Dicoumarin, 104; dicumarol, 90; heparin, 4, 90, 103-104

Blood, whole, transfusions, 18, 19

Blue Cross, 255, 261

Blue Shield, 255, 261

Bone grafts, 213, 215

Brain injuries, ambulant treatment, 169-170; dehydrating, 167, 168; drainage, 167; operations, 165, 166; plasma injections, 168

Brooks, B., 129

Buerger's Disease, 126

Burns, 196-207

Burns, treatment for, "Bundling for Burns," 197, 204-207; débridement, 201, 204; penicillin, 203, 207; skin grafting, 205-206, 207; sulfadiazine, 202; tannic acid spray, 198; transfusions, 197, 200

Bursitis, 186

Cancer, 227-240; bone, 230; breast, 229-230, 234-235, 236; cervix, 239; colon, 238; epidermoid, 234; facial, 234; intestinal, 231, 236; liver, 231, 232; lungs, 239; pancreas, 85-86, 240; prostate, 230-231; rectal, 237, 239; skin, 234; stomach, 236-239; uterus, 239

Cancer, treatment; operative anesthesia, 87; operative procedure, 87-88; preoperative preparation, 87; radium, 228; surgery, 228; X-rays, 228

Cardiac tamponade, 105

Carrel-Dakin solution, 46, 54

Cartilage grafts, 213, 215

Chain, E., 39-40

Chloroform, in anesthesia, 20-21; in childbirth, 21; effect on liver, 21, 71

Chloromycetin, 42

Chloropromazine, 178

Cineplastic amputation, 216-217

Circulation, anatomoses, 117; autonomic nervous system, 118; pulmonary, 117; systemic, 117

Clinics, group, 256-258

Clostridia bacillus, 50, 51, 54; sources of, 50-53

Cocoanut Grove disaster, 197, 206

Cold, effects on the body, 129

Colitis, 222

Colloids, 5, 11, 12; osmotic pressure of, 11, 12

Colorimeter, photoelectric, 4, 15

Colostomy, 239

Cortisone, 5, 9, 30, 200, 207, 252, 254

Costs of surgery, 241-248

Crawfoord, Clarence, 112

Crile, George, 188

Cryotherapy, 127-136; anesthesia for amputations, 129-130; anesthesia for diabetes, 129-130; anesthesia for minor operations, 128; ice caps for appendicitis, 128; use in trench foot, 132

Cushing, Harvey, 160, 169

Cyclopropane, 4, 23, 242

Cystic duct, 72, 73; artificial duct, 79-80

Dandy, Walter E., 164

Darwin, Charles, 21

Dees, John, 63-64

Degenerative diseases, 251-252

Dermatome (Padgett), 205, 208, 214, 215

Dextran, 200, 207

d'Harcourt, Colonel J. H., 47, 49

D'Herelle, Felix, 33

Diabetes, 71, 83, 84; diabetic coma, 84; diabetic convulsions, 84; during pregnancy, 89; surgery, 84; treatment, 89; with "cold" anesthesia, 128

Dicoumarin, 104, 120, 158

Dicumarol, 90

Domagk, Gerhard, 35

Duncan, G. W., 129

Ehrlich, Paul, 42

Electric shock, in mental diseases, 172

Electrocardiogram, 3

Electrocardiograph, 189, 242

Embryona, 229

Empyema, 94, 95, 96, 98, 100; first aid, 100

Endocrine glands, formation, 82; study of, 252

Ether, anesthesia, 22; effect on lungs, 22; preparation, 22

Facial injuries, treatment, acrylic dental splint, 208; facial moulage, 208, 216; fixation for fractured jaws, 208, 211, 212; plastic surgery, 208-216; repairing nose defects, 212; split-skin grafts, 208

Falling-drop apparatus, 15, 16, 200

Fallot, Etienne-Louis Arthur, 110

Fauteux, Mercier, 114

Fay, Temple, 127

Femoral thrombophlebitis, see Phlebitis

Fibrillation, 30-31

Field Surgery in Total War, 47

Firsts, operation on coronary artery, 3; patch on the heart, 5

Fleming, Alexander, 33-35, 39

Florey, H. W., 39-40

Fluoroscope, 3, 4, 242

Fractures, treatment, 9; use of metal nails, 189; Primer on Fractures, 9

Freeman, Walter J., 174

Frostbite, 129, 133; treatment, 135

Galileo, 21

Gall bladder, infection, 72; removal, 78, 79; surgery, 73, 76-79; use, 72

Gallstones, formation, 72; escape, 73

Gangrene, from diabetes, 131; from tourniquets, 131; in trench foot, 134-135

Gas gangrene, 10, 45, 47, 49-56, 62; cause, 53-54; germs carried by clothes, 50; in facial wounds, 209; prevention of, 54-55; symptoms, 51-52

Gastroscope, 237

Geriatrics, 252

Globulin, protection of antibodies, 18

Glycogen, 70

Gold, in cleft palates, 189

Grafts, bone, 213; cartilage, 213, 215; homografts, 89; isografts, 89; skin, 88, 89, 205, 206, 213-216

Gross, Robert E., 109, 112

Halstead, William H., 235

Heart, knife wounds, 104-105; operations, 2; war wounds, 106

Hematoma, 121, 122; pulsating, 121-122, 160

Hemoconcentration, 7

Hemoglobin, carried by, 10; determination of values, 4; lack of, 116, 117; reduced, 7

Hemorrhage, control, 66; in facial injuries, 209, 211; in liver operations, 75; treatment, 65-66; with shock, 65

Heparin, 4, 90, 103-104, 120, 158

Hippocrates, 197

Holmes, Oliver Wendell, 21

Homans, John, 155, 156

Hunter, William, 110

Hyperthyroidism, 82, 253

Hypothermia, 128

I^{131}, 253

Ileus, adynamic, 59-64, 67, 68

Immersion foot, 129; cause, 132-135; treatment, see Trench foot

Immunization, tetanus toxoid, 55

Infection, conquest of, 5

Infection, protection against, sulfa drugs, 5; penicillin, 5; "-mycin" group, 5

Infections, parasitic, 249; virus, 92-93, 233, 249

Influenza, 93-95

Insulin, 70, 71, 83, 84, 88; use in mental disease, 84, 172

Islands of Langerhans, 83, 85, 88, 90

Jacobsen, Carlyle, 173

Jaundice, cause, 74, 86; operations, 73, 74, 75, 76; painless, 86, 87; treatment, 76-77

Jolly, Major Douglas W., 47

Joubert, J. F., 33

Kolletschka, 32

Lahey Clinic, 256

Laminectomy, 162

Lane, Sir William Arbuthnot, 189

Larrey, Baron, 132

Larrey, Dominique Jean, 44

Lister, Joseph, 45, 172, 189

Liver, de-animation, 71; filtration plant, 70; indispensable organ, 69; storehouse for sugar, 70; surgery, 69, 79-80

Lobule, digestive function, 72; failure to act, 74; use, 70

Loew, Otto, 39

Long, Crawford, 22

Lundy, John S., 25

Lyerly, James G., 174

Lymph nodes, 230, 231, 235, 236, 238

Magnesium, in fractures, 190

Marsupialization, 85

Matas, Rudolph, 122

Mayo Clinic, 25, 256

Mediastinum, 96, 97; flutter, 96-97

Medicine, in Atomic Age, 249-258

Meningitis, 250-251

Metabolism machines, 242

Metastasis, 86, 127, 230, 231, 234

Metrazol, 172

Mickulicz operation, 238-239

Microtome, freezing, 242

Miller-Abbott Tube, 61-62, 67-68, 238

Moniz, Egas, 173-174

Morton, Thomas, 22

Moulage, facial, 208, 216

Nervous system, autonomic, 219-221; description of, 161-162; injuries to, 162-165

Neuritis, 186

Novocain, anesthesia, 29; brain surgery, 175; phlebitis, 152, 153

Ochsner, Alton, 158

Oligemia, 199

Operations, safety, 148-159

Orr, Winnet, 46

Oscillometer, 242

Osmotic pressure, 11, 12, 167

Oxygen, lack, 116-117, 131; tent, 5

Oxyhemoglobin, 7

P³², 253

Padgett, Earl C., 205, 208, 214

Pain, conquest of, 5

Painton, Lt. Col. Joseph F., 251

Pancreas, 81-90; cancer of, 86, 87; formation, 81, 82; function, 83-84; position, 81; surgery, 81, 84-86; transplanting, 88-89; tumors, 85

Papaverine, in vascular surgery, 121

Paré, Ambroise, 44, 45

Pasteur, Louis, 52, 53, 45, 172

Patent ductus arteriosus, 109-110; cause, 108-109; surgery, 109-110

Pectin, use in shock, 14

Pedicle flaps, 211

Penicillin, discovery, 33-40; use in abdominal wounds, 66; use in burns, 203, 207; use in chest wounds, 101; use in facial injuries, 210; use in gas gangrene, 55; use in gonorrhea, 41; use in postwar medicine, 250; use in staphylococcus, 34, 35; use in streptococcus, 35; use in syphilis, 41-42; structural formula, 40

Pentothal, aid in dressing wounds, 27; anesthesia, 25-28; use in head wounds, 27; use in tumors, 236

Pericarditis, cause and treatment, 106, 107

Peripheral vasoconstriction, 13

Peritonitis, 58-68; causes, 58, 59, 62; treatment, 59-65

Petronius, 189

Phlebitis, symptoms, 150, 151; treatment, 150-154

Phlebography, 156

Phonocardiogram, 3

Pickrell, Kenneth L., 202

Plan for medical care, 259-261

Plasma, constituents, 11; processing, 16-17; separation, 10, 16; use in abdominal wounds, 66, 67; use in brain injuries, 168; use in burns, 199, 200, 205, 206; use in facial injuries, 214

Pneumonia, following influenza, 94, 95

Pneumothorax, open, 96-101

Pneumothorax, tension, causes, 101; treatment, 101-102

Potts, Willis J., 111

Prefrontal lobotomy, 174-179

Primer on Fractures, 9

Prostheses appliances, 215-217

Prothrombin, formation, 74-75; measuring, 76, 77

Psychoneurosis, 221

Psychosurgery, 171-179; affective psychoses, 177; dementia praecox, 172; hysteria, 171; obsessive-compulsive neuroses, 173; schizophrenia, 178

Pudenz, Robert H., 193

Pulmonary embolus, 149, 150, 153-159

Quick, A. J., 76

Radioactive isotopes, gold, 254; iodine, 253; phosphorus, 253

Reed, Walter, 63

Reserpine, 178

Respiratory infections, preventive measures, 91, 92; vaccines, 93

Sacroiliac, *see* Sciatica

Salk vaccine, 18

Sano, M. E., 214

Sciatica, 180-187; hernia of the intervertebral disc, 184; operating procedure, 185-186

Semmelweis, Ignatz, 21, 32, 45, 203

Shock, conquest of, 5-19; cause, 8, 12-13, 18; control, 26; in burns, 197-198, 199, 200; in war injuries, 66; symptoms, 6-8; treatment, 14, 15, 16

Shock, neurogenic, 198

Silver, in surgery, 189-190

Simpson, Sir James Y., 21

Skin grafts, 88, 89; homografts, 89; in burns, 205, 206, 213-216; isografts, 89

Smithy, Horace G., 114

Spasms, in blood vessels, 120, 149, 152

Spinal column, construction, 183, 184

Spinal fluid, formation, 164, 165; drainage, 167

Spurling, Lt. Col. R. G., 193

Stainless steel, in bone injuries, 190

Staphylococcus, 33-35

Stimulants, Metrazol, 25

Streptomycin, 42

Suffocation, in facial injuries, 210, 211

Sulfa drugs, sulfadiazine, 36, 39, 67, 250-251; sulfaguanidine, 238; sulfanilamide, 36-38, 62-65, 67, 201-203, 210; sulfapyridine, 36-38; Sulfasuxadine, 238; sulfathiazole, 36, 39

Sulfadiazine, 39; in meningitis, 250, 251; in open wounds, 67; in prophylaxis, 250, 251; in respiratory infections, 251

Sulfaguanidine, 238

Sulfanilamide, 36; in battle wounds, 37; in burns, 201-203; in facial injuries, 210; in peritonitis, 62-65, 67; in pneumonia, 38; in streptococcus, 36

Sulfapyridine, against pneumococcus, 38

Sulfasuxadine, 238

Sulfathiazole, against gonococcus, 39; against meningococcus, 39; against pneumococcus, 39; against staphylococcus, 39; against streptococcus, 39

Surgeon, cost of training, 244-245; how to choose a surgeon, 246-247

Surgery, adequate, 54, 56; antiseptic, 45, 46; closed plaster, 46, 47, 52; early, 54, 56; heart, 103-115; in war, 47-49; plastic and maxillofacial, 208-217; psychosomatic, 218-226

Surgery, chest, 91-102; with intratracheal tubes, 99, 100

Surgery, costs of, 241-248

Surgery, vascular, 116-126; by amputation, 118-119; by ice packs, 121; by novocain injections, 121; by tying off, 120-121

Surgery in war, 47-57; casualty classification, 47, 48; Collecting Stations, 47; no substitute, 56; Special Base Hospitals, 48

Tannic acid, see Burns, treatment for

Tantalum, 188-195; discovery, 191; method of using, 192-194; physical properties, 192; use in electronics, 192; use in facial injuries, 213, 215

Taussig, Helen A., 110, 111

Terramycin, 42

Tetra-bromphenolphthalein, use with X-ray, 76

That None Should Die, 258-261

Thermocouples, 242

Thiouracil, 253

Thrombin, 74

Thrombosis, 103

Thyroid gland, 82

Touroff, Arthur S. W., 109

Transfusions, in abdominal wounds, 66; in liver operations, 67; in pancreas operations, 87

Treatment of War Wounds and Fractures, 47

Trench foot, 129; cause, 132-135; symptoms, 135; treatment, 132-135

Trepine, 160

Trueta, J., 47, 49, 52, 54, 56

Trypsin, 82, 84, 85, 90

Tumors, adenomas, 232; benign, 232, 236; breast, 234-236; lipomas, 232

2-methyl-1, 4 naphthoquinone, 75

Ulcers, stomach, 221, 237

Ultraviolet lamps, use of, 4

Valerius Cordus, 22

Vanadium steel, in bone surgery, 190

Varicose eczema, 137, 142; *see also* Varicose veins

Varicose ulcer, 137, 142; treatment, 145-146; *see also* Varicose veins

Varicose veins, 137-147; formation, 137-141; heredity, 141; in pregnancy, 141; position, 137-142; treatment, 142-145

Vasospasm, 119, 120

Venable, Charles S., 190, 192

Venography, 156

Vitallium, in bladder surgery, 79; in bone injuries, 190-191; in vascular surgery, 120

Vitamin K, 74-77, 79, 87

Von Bolton, Werner, 191

Waksman, Selman A., 42

Watts, James W., 174

Welch, Claude E., 237

Welch bacillus, 10, 49-50, 52, 54, 62

Whipple, Allen O., 87

Wounds, early treatment, 56

Wry neck, 186

*"An unsurpassed tale
of devotion..."*

THE SONG OF RUTH

by Frank G. Slaughter

The memorable love story of the Bible's most beautiful heroine is told by one of the greatest novelists of our time. *The Song of Ruth* will live in your heart forever.

Now Available — PERMABOOK M-4031——35¢

The real story of real war—

TO HELL AND BACK

by Audie Murphy
America's Most Decorated Soldier

A great story of guns, guts and teamwork in the
infantry during World War II. This book was a
best seller in the higher-priced edition and became an
outstanding movie with the author in the starring role.
A famous story that will live long in the memory
of all who read it.

Now Available — PERMABOOK M-4029 — 35¢